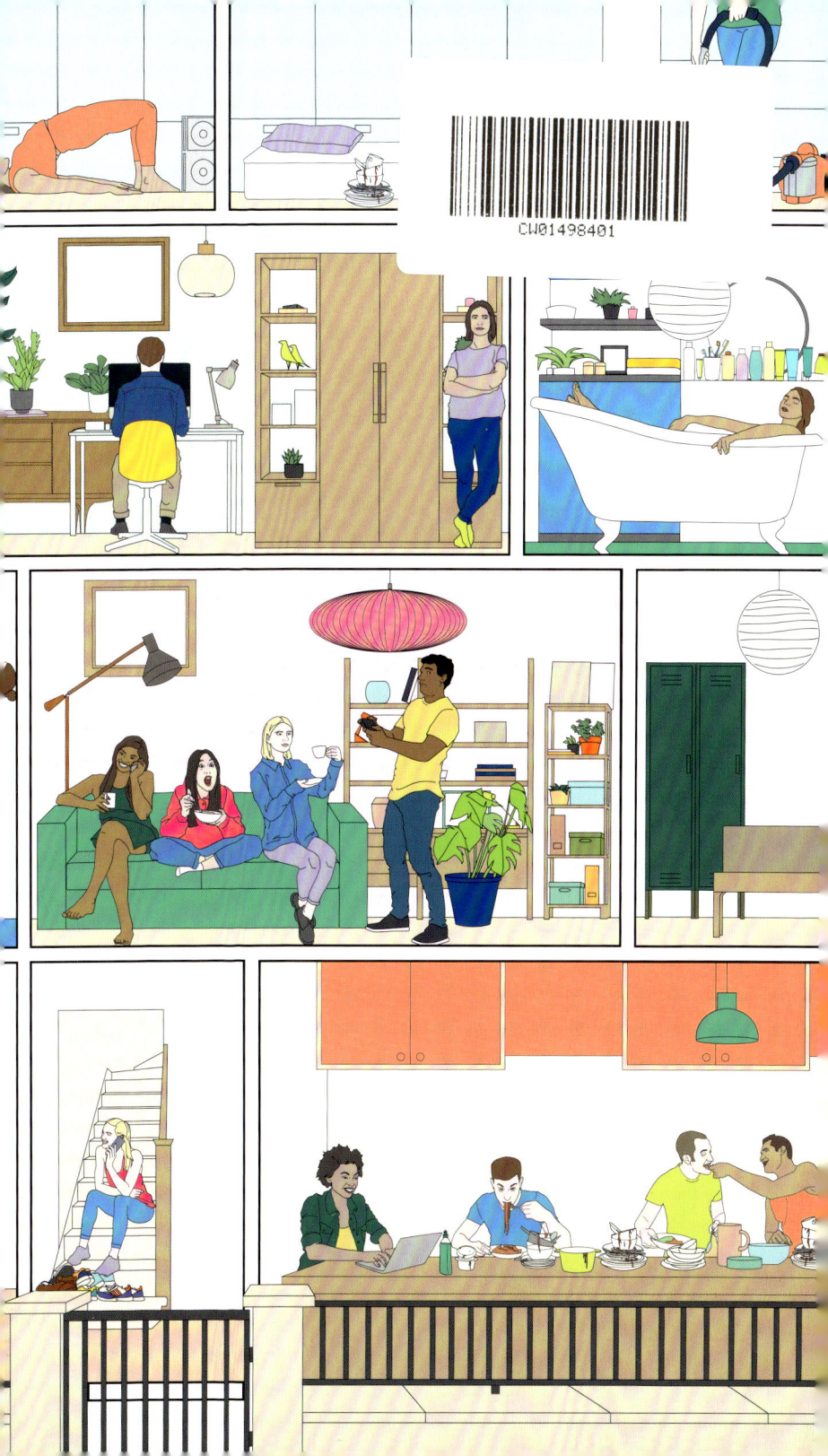

HOW
TO
STAY
SANE
IN A
HOUSE
SHARE

HOW TO STAY SANE IN A HOUSE SHARE

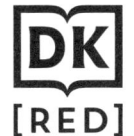

Alice Wilkinson

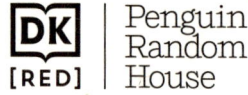

First published in Great Britain in 2025 by
DK RED, an imprint of
Dorling Kindersley Limited
20 Vauxhall Bridge Road,
London SW1V 2SA

The authorised representative in the EEA is
Dorling Kindersley Verlag GmbH. Arnulfstr. 124,
80636 Munich, Germany

A CIP catalogue record for this book
is available from the British Library.
PB ISBN: 978-0-2416-9634-7

Printed and bound in the United Kingdom

www.dk.com

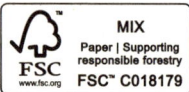

This book was made with Forest
Stewardship Council™ certified
paper – one small step in DK's
commitment to a sustainable future.
Learn more at **www.dk.com/uk/
information/sustainability**

ADVANCE PRAISE FOR
HOW TO STAY SANE IN A HOUSE SHARE

'A brilliantly researched and compelling read. It tackles an area of
relationships that has so far been overlooked and combines deep
psychological thinking with practical advice and takeaways.'
Emma Reed Turrell

'A brilliant look at modern womanhood through the relatable,
Big Roasting Tin, bath mat, broken boiler lens of house shares.'
Nell Frizzell

'Kind, wise and genuinely useful – this book is an essential
guide to modern living, and hugely comforting too.'
Daisy Buchanan

'A deeply insightful, practical and sensitive exploration
of the housing crisis and what it means to live in a house share
today. Alice has crafted this book from a place of personal
experience, backed up by research and science, the resulting
book should be required reading for all house sharers.'
Rosie Kellett

'This is a comprehensive, thoughtful guide that provides much-
needed practical advice but crucially a vital sense of optimism.
A timely helping hand!'
Yomi Adegoke

'Alice Wilkinson serves as a wise and empathetic guide to one of
the most unexamined yet fraught aspects of millennial life. But she
also goes deeper, exploring themes that are central to a life well
lived: the importance of self examination, how to set boundaries,
and finding connection in a disconnected world.'
Rosie Spinks

'A love letter to home and friendship and a damning
indictment of our housing crisis.'
Kieran Yates

'This a first-of-its-kind look at what is right in front of so many
of us. It takes in all of the joy and misery of the way modern
women often live today and deftly engages with how space –
both personal and political – comes from where we rest
and how we share those vulnerable moments.'
Sophie Wilkinson

Contents

Introduction   **10**

1. **A room of her own:** why so many women
   are house sharing   **16**

2. **Meeting point:** how to choose
   (good) housemates   **38**

3. **Peas in a pod:** living with friends
   and how to do it well   **62**

4. **Rupture and repair:** how to handle
   housemate conflicts   **86**

5. **The pecking order:** housemate hierarch
   and how to find harmony   **112**

6. **Rental health:** managing mental wellbeing
   in a house share   **138**

7. **Precious things:** the role of our belonging
   in belonging   **162**

8. **Dating by committee:** boundaries
   and benefits of dating in a house share   **180**

9. **It's time:** shutting the door on
   a house share   **206**

Conclusion   **230**

Acknowledgements   **234**
Notes   **236**
Select bibliography   **252**
About the author   **254**

For Lucy and Laura – permanent fixtures in all my homes

Introduction

The weeks before I broke up with my boyfriend, Noah,* my mind was whirring with hazy projections about what life would be like. Dismantling our two-and-a-half-year relationship meant leaving the one-bed flat that we lived in together. Of all the fears that consumed me on the brink of being single at 32, living in a house share again terrified me the most.

Three years earlier I'd matched with Noah on Bumble during a bout of dating app doomswiping, lying in my bed in my shared house in Balham, London, where I was living with three others. I was 29, eager to progress in life and I was acutely aware that because of the rising cost of living, meeting a partner might be the only ticket out of shared living. My house sharing status fired up the same kind of blinding determination I'd felt when I was an intern, yet wanting to be a writer.

I was in a house share, but I wanted my own place. It became a fixation that infiltrated every aspect of my being. I was furiously clambering the career ladder because better pay would mean I had a better chance of affording somewhere of my own. Every time a friend managed it – as so many were starting to do approaching 30 – I felt a pang of intense jealousy followed by sheer panic that I wasn't getting where I wanted to be fast enough.

'Lost', 'stuck', and 'rootless' are the words I'd use time and time again to describe my feelings during those house sharing years. 'Lost' because it wasn't the life I'd seen for myself. 'Stuck' because nothing had prepared me for dealing with the plethora of personalities and conflicts that arise in a house share. 'Rootless' because, as housemates and house shares rotated around me, I longed for a place that stayed still, one I could nurture and invest in. At that point, I'd lived with 17 different housemates (plus a rabbit) in seven different house shares and I romanticised what it would be like not to live in one.

---

* His name has been changed, like the names of others in this book. But all the stories are true.

When I fell in love with Noah, things moved quickly. In part, I think this was fuelled by my burning desire to make a home of my own – not one that I shared with people I'd met on SpareRoom. After six months of dating, we moved in to a rented place, just us. I skipped out the door of that Balham house share, giddy with excitement about having a whole (albeit small) kitchen full of cupboards to fill and choices that would be ours alone to make, no housemates to consider.

By the time I was 30, it looked as though I had all my ducks in a row: a committed partner, a flat we shared, a job I liked. But there was an emptiness. I'd longed so much for my own place and now I had it. I'd take huge pleasure in having the space and feeling the calmness of not needing to consider three others' lives. But then I'd sit in the quiet of our flat and miss my housemates – the connection, the support, the hilarity. I missed discussing work conundrums that only other females would get, I missed sharing bottles of wine on random Thursday evenings, I missed asking them for their opinions on my outfit or borrowing a pair of tights when I discovered, last minute, all mine were laddered.

Feeling 'stuck in a house share' is all-encompassing. That 29-year-old version of me – fed up with the low-level tension that's ever-present in a house share and completely fixated on getting out – never thought there might be aspects I'd miss about it. But there were. I missed my housemates. I missed hearing their news, getting to taste their culinary experiments, being invited along to exhibitions that I'd never think to go to, exercise classes I wasn't brave enough to try alone. I had been more outward-looking, connected and inspired then.

In that two-year sabbatical from house sharing when I lived with Noah, it slowly dawned on me what I'd walked away from when I left that last house share. In those early days of our relationship, I loved living with him but, still, I had a niggle that I'd rushed into it, not fully savouring the house share I was soon to leave behind. My desire to progress had stopped me from feeling connected, grounded, and 'at home' there. I hadn't allowed myself to appreciate how precious it was.

House shares always seemed temporary to me. The people I was living with and places I was living in were stopgaps – relationships and addresses I'd be in for just a year or two before I got on with the rest of my life. When that temporary stopgap became 10 years and counting of living in house shares, I knew I needed to change mindset. Because, today, we are living in house shares for a significant proportion of our adult lives.

And yet there is a dearth of advice on how to make house sharing work for you. In a world of TikTok therapy and psychology influencers, we hear the impact romantic relationships, friendships, and family have on our mental wellbeing. We're taught terminology and coping mechanisms that help us to deal with challenges that arise. Despite the fact we live in very close quarters with housemates, often for years, potentially building very intimate relationships with them, barely anyone tells us how to handle housemate relationships well. And in my experience, house sharing is a blind spot among my parents' generation too. They can offer advice in the arena of romantic relationships and friendships to a point, but draw a blank at housemates. Their generation didn't live in house shares for as long as we do today.

That lack of guidance, conversation, and advice only exacerbates the feeling of being stuck in a house share when we face frustrations, conflicts, and situations we're not equipped with the language to understand or the tools to resolve. Perhaps if we were, we wouldn't feel so stuck. Perhaps knowing how to deal with the frustrations that arise would allow us to enjoy all the connections and opportunities that house sharing offers.

This book is my attempt at closing those wisdom gaps for you in a way that I wish someone had for me. I asked myself what it means to house share well and these are my findings. In the first chapter, I look at how history has shaped modern-day house sharing. Then, I explore how we can house share better. From how to meet a 'good' housemate to handling conflict and dating in a house share, you'll find anecdotes from my own house shares, practical advice, and reflections at the end of each chapter to help you work through scenarios that might be happening in your living space.

I started researching this book three days after I ended my relationship with Noah. Armed with the skills I'd honed during a decade in journalism, I began writing something that was closer to my heart than anything I'd worked on before. I unlocked my SpareRoom account, which had been stagnant for years, and felt that lost and rootless feeling creep back in. It took me a few months to find a new house share. But in the weeks and months that followed the break-up, I started visiting and chatting to the women living in house shares who are featured in this book. Instead of the nightmares and tales of woe that I'd been fully prepared to hear – and of which there were, of course, some – most of the women wanted to share how nurturing their house shares had been.

I came away from those conversations reminded of how powerful it can be to share a space with other women who are on the same path as you. I listened to stories of housemates supporting one another, the ways they made space for everyone's anxieties and quirks. The little kindnesses that lifted people up when they needed it. The feelings of connection they shared. I heard memories of power cuts and floods, when they'd pulled together, spontaneous cocktail nights they'll remember for years to come, lifelong friendships formed over weeknight dinners, hanging one another's laundry up, and chats waiting for the kettle to boil.

So I re-entered my house sharing years afresh. In my eighth house share with my 18th housemate, I'm doing things differently. I'm cherishing the connection and discovering for myself that I can feel at home in a shared space when I face up to the frustrations and challenges and know how to navigate them. It is possible to stay sane, live harmoniously – and even thrive – in a house share. This book is my take on how.

1. A room of her own

Why so many women
are house sharing

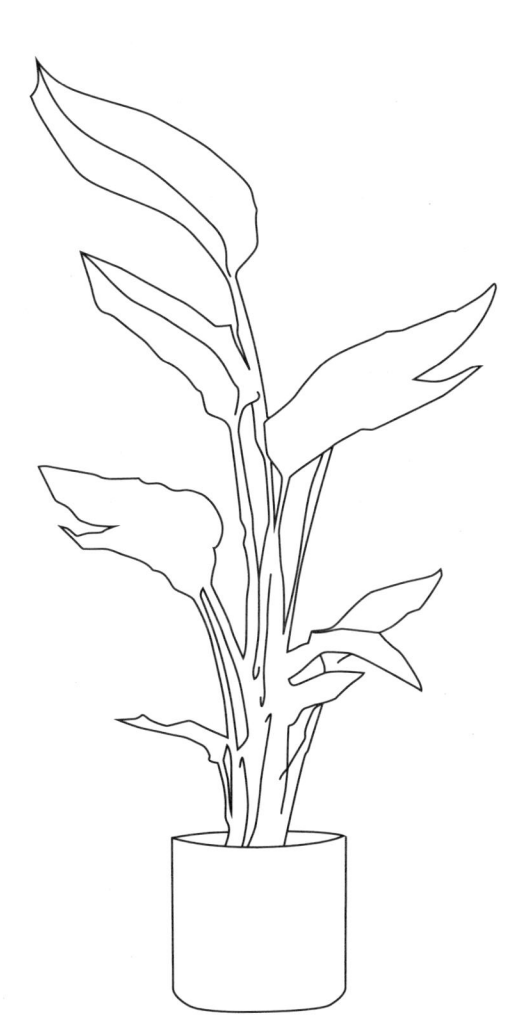

"For we think back through our
mothers if we are women"
Virginia Woolf[1]

My eyes well up when I open the fridge door. The Big Roasting Tin is sitting there, full to the brim with a rice salad that my housemate, Phoebe, made last night. In any other scenario, it might have been a nice surprise, but it's been one of those weeks and living in a house share is getting on top of me.

I'm 28 at this point and an editor at a magazine, yet I can't find a clean T-shirt because of a backlog of clothes needing to be washed as the machine is always full with other people's loads. I'm approaching a big deadline at work and craving some solitude in the evenings, but each day this week, one or two of my housemates have had friends or partners over. And we all did a big food shop at the weekend, so our fridge, freezer, and cupboards are bursting at the seams. I have to play food Tetris just to get a teabag.

With only five kitchen cupboards between us, we don't have the room to duplicate kitchen items. That's how the Big Roasting Tin – the largest oven dish I own – became a house favourite. I'd bought it because it's the same as my mum's: a large, rectangular, white enamel tray with a blue rim. Hers was the centrepiece at mealtimes throughout my childhood, so mine indulges my nostalgia for the home I grew up in. I'd always thought it was a given that by 25 I'd be a working mother living in domestic wedded bliss, serving dinner from a tin like this on to the plates of my growing children. Instead, I turned 25, then 26, then 27, then 28, and my hard-to-break enamelware has weathered seven different flats and served dishes cooked in it to 17 different housemates. Now, the shared tin goes in and out of the oven several times a day, holding food cooked by me or one of the three women I live with before being dished out between an ever-changing combination of housemates plus attached partners.

The present company determines the vibe in the kitchen on any given evening. Phoebe plus Jess means I can tell them I had a shit day, offload a bit, and sulk unapologetically while cooking. Phoebe plus boyfriend plus quieter housemate, Sophie, usually means slightly forced chat as – between making the necessary noises to politely and awkwardly make my way round a shared kitchen at dinner time – I try to make conversation that addresses everyone.

'Hi, Ben. How's things? Sorry, can I just squeeze behind you to put my milk in the fridge?'

'Phoebe, do you mind if I chuck out the dregs of your orange juice? It's smelling a bit vinegary. I've just bought some new that I need to squeeze into the door – you can help yourself.'

'Ah, sorry to be annoying, Sophie – can I just borrow this end of your chopping board to slice my onion, sorry. What's the knife been used for? Thanks so much! Sorry.'

It's a rare but fun occurrence when we eat together just us four housemates (without partners). Even rarer and more fun is when no one else is in. I'll play a podcast out loud, make space in the communal fridge for my shopping, and have free rein of the utensils, appliances... and the Big Roasting Tin.

So that Monday evening, I arrived home from work and, as always, paused for a few seconds at the bottom of the stairs, listening to check who was home before making my entrance. Silence meant space. I hadn't noticed that my neck and shoulder muscles were so tense until I felt them let go. I knew then that I could unwind while cooking my chorizo chicken bake, putting the day's stresses to the back of my mind. Let the peelings scatter all over the worktop, use multiple chopping boards, pile the washing-up in the sink, and deal with it after I'd eaten.

But the Big Roasting Tin being full of my housemate's food in the fridge is a problem.

The panicked breathing starts when I'm sitting on the kitchen floor, crying on the phone to my mum. The cupboard handles dig into my back while I stare at the flakes of onion skin and ends of spaghetti on the floor. In between short, sharp whimpers, I respond to my mum's concerned questioning on the phone: 'Oh, Ally, take some deep breaths. Come on. Can you say what's upsetting you?' I'm in full flow, telling her how the tin that I wanted to use to cook my dinner in is full of someone else's food when I catch a glimpse of myself through her eyes. I wonder, too, why I'm reacting to this so intensely. But then my mum suggests pan-frying the chicken thighs instead and I hang up, abandon my cooking, pad up the stairs to my room, press the door shut, and sob into my pillow. I let the existential rage take hold.

This isn't about the tin.

It's the hour I spend on my daily commute home worrying about who'll be in the kitchen when I get back. It's having to ask permission from the household every time I want to have friends over for dinner or family to stay. It's the open forum on who I'm dating and where we're at – after date two. It's the four-way discussions about what we watch on TV. It's negotiating with three other women as to whose pile of washing will go into the machine first. And it's 10 years' worth of sharing houses where the nice bath mat I'd bought a week before just 'disappeared', finding my new white Arket T-shirt stained and on my housemate's bedroom floor, her boyfriend stashing his MDMA in a jar next to where we keep our teabags. It's waking up to period blood in the toilet, finding fragments of my favourite mug in the bin, lying awake listening to giggly sex until 3am while my own love life is in bits. Dinner plates growing mould under the sofa, bumping into my housemate's one-night stand naked on the landing. Trying to pursue a career while fielding the 35+ passive-aggressive WhatsApps in the house chat.

If you're house sharing, or have ever house shared, you'll no doubt have your own list of crimes committed.

For me right now, in my seventh house share, not being able to use my Big Roasting Tin is a sharp reminder that I am nowhere near where I want to be at 28. And as my house sharing years stretch out ahead of me, I'm riddled with homesickness for the roots I thought I'd have by now. Only 'homesickness' doesn't feel like the right term as there is no actual home to pin my yearning to. I read somewhere about the German word 'Fernweh' and wonder if it captures these feelings more accurately. It translates as 'far sickness', which is an ache and longing for a distant place you've never been. The definition feels more fitting because longing for something is painful. But longing for something that's intangible – in my case, a home that's hard to visualise and feels beyond my reach – is especially torturous.

I now know – after chatting with those I interviewed for this book and countless conversations with friends – that I'm not alone in having this feeling. And yet, five years on, as I continue on my house sharing journey, Big Roasting Tin in hand, there has been one life-altering shift when it comes to my living situation: my outlook.

Having taken a holistic approach to remedy my far sickness, I can see that it is a natural by-product of a punishing housing market combined with my own preconceptions of what a 'home' should look like. From what I can tell, there is a whole generation of people like me who, fed up with feeling 'stuck' in a house share, are desperate to know how they can do it better.

Before we can learn to navigate the challenges of the modern house share, it's helpful to look at and understand the external factors at play. In this chapter, we'll take a closer look at how, as a society, we've arrived at a point where we are house sharing for longer. Contextualising today's house sharing landscape like this can help us to realise that, as house sharers, we are not alone in the challenges we face.

No place like home

As a privileged, middle-class, white woman, spending my disposable income on Arket T-shirts and enamel roasting tins with blue rims, I'll never know what it's like not to be able to afford a roof over my head. But I am part of an ever-expanding community of professionals united by the endurance sport that is house sharing. I experience both the fun and the fury of it alongside 4.5 million people in the UK[2] and 1.79 million in the USA.[3] It's predicted that, in 2025, 7.2 million households in the UK will be in rented accommodation, which is a rise from 5.4 million in 2015.[4] With more than half of adults under the age of 40 expected to live in landlord-owned properties by 2025,[5] my community will be welcoming plenty more into its fold.

History tells us (and period dramas show us), that men were the 'breadwinners' and the property owners. They are no longer the only ones. Young women today value owning their own house more than having a partner or being married according to one survey undertaken in 2023.[6] However, as house prices increased by 207 per cent between 2000 and 2020,[7] 37 per cent of people in a poll undertaken in the UK in 2016 said home ownership 'will remain out of their reach for good'.[8] So house sharing is the only option for many people, particularly women, who nonetheless dream of having their own home. No doubt they're experiencing the same far sickness as me. It's a story we're seeing more and more. In 2021, SpareRoom reported having more people searching for rooms than they had rooms available.[9]

It's the state of human evolution in the 21st century: we work for more pay to get more space. Maybe you're on this path with me, striving for a better-paid job to earn enough money to afford your own place. My sense is that having a home of my own would grant me more agency and control over my life. I had a small taste of what it was like living outside of a house share and now, as a professional adult, I crave it more than ever. Perhaps, you too, are at a place in your life where you want to choose who enters your space and when, how it looks, how warm it is, how often to clean it, how loud you have the radio, whether to get a pet. To sing in the shower if you feel like it, organise your food in *all* the cupboards (not just the one you're allotted), walk around naked. Growing up, I assumed that I'd follow the same order of life stages that I'd observed most of the generation above me go through. I'd leave my family home, move to student accommodation, then a house share and, after a few years, get a place of my own.

But with today's housing market ensuring that the cost of buying a home has risen faster than our pay, you might be left wondering how individuals in our parents' generation managed to afford a house when we can't. Well, during the 1970s, the average price of a house was £9,277. That was 4.1 times the average annual income in that decade.[10] For us, in 2023, the average house price was £290,000.[11] That's 8.8 times the average annual income. Double what it was during the 1970s. The housing market is a very different place for us than it was for our parents.

The statistics get more alarming if you're a woman, thanks to the gender pay gap. The average annual income for a woman in the UK in 2023 was £31,672 and £37, 382 for a man.[12] A disparity you might already feel acutely in your own life. The average house price in the UK is almost 10 times the average woman's annual income.[13] And in London, it's 14 times that. When you look at these numbers, it's no wonder so many of us feel very far away from being able to own a home. It's because we are – 10 or 14 times our annual income away. Yet, as recently as 1999, the average house price in the UK was six times[14] the average woman's annual income, which then was £14,598.[15] It was only four times the average man's income for that year. The same is happening in the USA as houses are skyrocketing at a rate that is not being matched by incomes.[16]

The first step – saving enough money for a house deposit – feels just as unreachable. In 2023, the average time it took people to save a deposit[17] was nearly 10 years – longer for those with lower levels of pay. Again, that hasn't always been the case. In 1999, the deposit required was less than half the average household income in the UK.[18] But in 2023, the deposit for an average homebuyer is twice their annual income.[19]

At the time of writing this book, the average woman's annual income was 16 per cent less than that of the average for a man, but she spends a higher proportion of her pay on rent,[20] saving 35 per cent less than him on average.[21] More than a quarter of all renters are aged 35 or over,[22] and there's not a single region in England where it's affordable to rent in the private market on women's median earnings.[23] It makes sense, then, that more women who have not bought a property feel stressed that they'll be renting for the rest of their lives than men do in this group – 45 per cent of women compared with 39 per cent of men.[24] A rising population, not enough new homes, tighter lending rules, plus a cocktail of political moves have led us to a point where affording our own property seems an impossible feat for the average 30-something. It's stopping young professional women like me from feeling like we're making that final step we want to into adulthood and, with it, destabilising our sense of home and belonging.

Friends of mine who left house shares to rent alone are now

having to re-enter them as the cost-of-living crisis that began in late 2021 in the UK has hit women harder than men.[25] Others, like me, have re-entered them after the breakdown of a relationship, not able to afford to live alone. It's unsurprising that it's female voices we hear describing being 'stuck' in house shares. And yet, these are often impressive people with impressive jobs, stripped of agency and control the minute they enter the front door of their own homes. I've lived with directors of communication, accountants who lead teams of 30, event managers in charge of million-pound budgets, and biomedical scientists working on life-changing drugs. Being a career-driven young professional in a house share is an incongruous existence.

High-flyers in house shares

At the peak of my five-year stint working at a creative agency, I was the editor of a health magazine. When the agency pitched to potential new clients, it was me they'd call on to play the role of resident wellbeing expert and present their ideas. On the day of one particular pitch, feeling pressure to win the business for the agency, I dressed the part and walked into the meeting. I adopted a persona: cool, calm, knowledgeable, and professional. The presentation went well and I got pats on the back from my team. Recovering from the adrenaline rush, I got back to my desk and checked my phone. A string of WhatsApp notifications had stacked up in the house chat while I'd been presenting.

Jess: Guys, please stop piling the washing-up on the drainer. I'm trying to wash my dishes and there's nowhere for me to put them. Also, whose turn is it to buy cleaning stuff? We need bleach and washing-up liquid.

Phoebe: I bought that last month so must be Alice or Sophie?? xxxxx

Sophie: I'll get it after work. So @Alice can you remember it's your turn next? x

A discussion ensued over who had piled their dishes on the drainer. Not present to defend myself, it was insinuated that I was the culprit. The professional persona I'd put on that day was immediately shattered to pieces by the 25 messages fired in the house WhatsApp chat. The responsibility and respect I'd been gaining as I progressed in my career undercut by the lack of agency I had over my home life in a house share.

In the eight house shares I've lived in with young professional women, the pressure to succeed in our careers is palpable. Research shows that women in the USA are becoming more career-driven than men, with 66 per cent of 18–34-year-old women citing a high-paying career among their top life priorities, compared with just 59 per cent of young men.[26] It makes sense to me that women have to prioritise a well-paid career in a way that men don't, and it is creating a workforce of ambitious young women driven by a genuine need to earn more to afford the same aspirational lifestyle that we see higher-earning men in the same industries accessing with greater ease. With women workers earning 80 per cent of what men earn[27] and a rate of progress that shows it will be 2069 before we get equal pay,[28] we are working harder and more – an hour longer than men each day according to the World Economic Forum[29] – to afford the agency over our own lives that comes with having a home of our own.

Belonging

'Home' means different things for each of us. But the beauty of having your own home is that you have the power to make it all the things you need it to be, to create a restorative environment. You can unwind to music you like, surround yourself with books and plants, paint the walls with calming shades or fluorescent, glow-in-the-dark colours, if that's what you want. A home, to me, is a familiar place where I can return to restore. Crucially, though, a home of my own would mean choosing who enters, exits, having a physical boundary that would allow me to protect my peace, and where the people around me are invested in making that space restorative for me, and me for them. It seems easier to achieve this in a family set-up or a romantic relationship where you care deeply about one another, share value systems, and future goals. A house share tests all the defining characteristics of what a home means – as the chapters that follow explore.

I see listings on SpareRoom by women who, just as I am, are 'looking for a housemate who wants to make their house a home' or housemates 'looking for a home that's a sanctuary'. This wording nods to an unspoken code that you're committing to making it a place where you look after one another, protect, and invest in the space. I wonder, though, whether a house share can ever feel like a sanctuary when, by its very nature, you are on different paths and planning separate futures. It's also a set-up that demands compromise: on how the space is used, making room for everyone's quirks and preferences, and respecting differences in order to live alongside one another.

Having lived with male and female housemates and listened to male friends talk about their house shares, I get the overwhelming sense that – while house sharing absolutely has impacts on all sexes and sexualities – the challenges of shared living hit women differently. The effects are deeper, somehow. When I see headlines about house sharing reference being 'stuck in a house share',[30] how they're 'a symptom of a bonkers property market',[31] and it 'actually makes you miserable',[32] I don't need to read the bylines to know that they were written by women. In so many ways, my generation has been granted choices the ones before us didn't have. I can conceive a child on my own, freeze my eggs, travel the world working as a digital nomad, retrain as a surgeon. But among all this choice, having my own home is not a freedom I can access. While 50 per cent of baby boomers in the UK, born less than 50 years before me, had their own place aged 30,[33] many millennials are struggling to do the same. Yet, 77 per cent of 25–39-year-olds and 83 per cent of 16–24-year-olds currently feel pressure to reach life's milestones, such as to buy a house, get married, and have children.[34] That pressure is only increased by an awareness that we're not reaching these milestones by the same ages as previous generations.

If house sharing makes me a woman of my time, my mum was a woman of hers – marrying at 22 and celebrating the arrival of her third child at 29 (the age I was when I celebrated the arrival of a third Big Roasting Tin). In the 1960s, 76 per cent of those getting married in England and Wales were under the age of 25, like my mum was. By 2012, times had changed and just 14 per cent of those getting married were under 25. Marriage rates decreased as much as 50 per cent between 1972 and 2019,[35] and while many couples are cohabiting, there is a general movement away from following tradition and living as married couples, which adds even more context to why so many of us are house sharing. I am one of the first generation of women in England and Wales in which more than half (50.1 per cent) turned 30 having had no children – a percentage that's more than doubled since 1941, when 17.9 per cent of women were child-free by the time they were 30.

In 1974 – the year my mum celebrated her 12th birthday – a new law was introduced that meant single or divorced women in the USA could apply for a mortgage without a man. By 1975, as my mum was turning 13, UK laws allowed women to open bank accounts and apply for credit and loans in their own name, and made it illegal to discriminate against women in the workplace.

When I was hosting a Forever Friends-themed 12th birthday party in 2003, J. K. Rowling was the best-paid author in the world and Sarah Jessica Parker was on the October cover of *Vogue*. She'd been on TV screens playing Carrie Bradshaw in *Sex and the City* for five years by then, epitomising what it meant to be a free woman – independent, single, living in her own place, and earning her own money. The pressures on me at 33 are so far removed from the ones that my mum had when she was my age, and the stark differences between our experiences as young women are never more obvious than when I turn to her for advice on housemate gripes.

I'd call my mum to vent my frustrations and ask for guidance on how to raise and resolve issues with my housemates, but she was often bemused at the situation I was in. The only solution we came up with between us was that I'd visit her for the weekend to get some space. It would provide some light relief, but it wasn't a solution that would bolster the foundations of my house share or be conducive to making the house share a happier place.

For me, my peers, and perhaps you, too, we are the first generation in a line of women in our families to be house sharing into our late 20s and 30s. This means our mothers either have limited lived experiences of it or none at all and can only go so far when offering advice. As a result, today's generation of professional young women are navigating uncharted waters, often without much support, as we face a unique set of challenges.

Turning full circle

Our parents' generation may not have house shared for as long as we do today, but house sharing is nothing new. While the following chapters interrogate what plays out inside the four walls of a modern house share, here, a potted history of house sharing provides an important backdrop to our current living situation.

Historically, women couldn't legally own property or the money they earned. It was only in 1848 in the USA, when the Women's Property Act was passed, and in 1870 in the UK, with the Married Women's Property Act[36] coming into force, that a woman could earn money in her own name and be a homeowner.

That was one of the first waves of feminism. Throughout history, the state of housing for women has been symbolic of the hardships or the freedoms they were being granted or denied elsewhere in society. It's why Jane Austen's female protagonists in *Pride and Prejudice* and *Sense and Sensibility,* unable to inherit their father's homes, needed to marry 'well'. As women challenged their traditional roles in the domestic sphere, where they were dependent on men, a house of their own became an emblem of what they were trying to achieve at the time: equal access to jobs, equal pay, and being able to earn enough to support themselves financially and live independently from men.

The First World War presented a window of opportunity for women regarding improving their position in the workplace and wider society. Two million women[37] joined the UK's workforce between 1914 and 1918 to do the jobs of the men who'd gone to fight, which meant that, while women had made up 24 per cent of the total number of people in employment in July 1914, this grew to 37 per cent by November 1918. In the USA, there were similar increases, women constituting 20 per cent[38] of the workforce in all manufacturing industries by the end of the First World War.

Women's lives were changing, but there wasn't the infrastructure to accommodate these changes. More women needed to live independently but, with landlords refusing to let properties to single women, they were forced to live in boarding houses and hostels.[39] Paving the way for many of us today, these women proved that they were capable of having careers outside those traditionally considered acceptable for women – but they were still being paid as much as half the money men would receive in the same roles.[40]

At the end of the war in 1918, there were 1.5 million more women than men in the UK. Those among them who were unlikely to marry and needed to support themselves financially became known as 'surplus women'. An article in the *Daily Mail* in 1921 read: 'The superfluous women are a disaster to the human race.'[41] These women, through no fault of their own, were ostracised from a society in which marriage still played a central role.

The tussle between the theoretical freedom that laws have granted women and the actual freedom their pay allows existed long before SpareRoom. In fact, it's existed for centuries,[42] as evidenced by the setting up of a number of women's organisations. The Women's Bureau was founded in the USA in 1920 to improve the welfare of women with jobs. The same year, Women's Pioneer Housing[43] was founded in the UK and, in 1934, the Over Thirty Association was set up to help the increasing number of single 'older' women to find employment and accommodation.

While formal barriers limiting women's freedom were slowly being removed, little was being done for the welfare of a single working woman being paid up to half as much as a man for doing the same job. On the one hand, laws were being passed that allowed women to live independently of men, own property, achieve an education, pursue careers outside the home, and find some financial freedom. On the other, they weren't being paid enough to support themselves – or to afford a home of their own.

For women who could live independently from men, the idea of home was changing but, still, their options were limited. In suffrage publications of the early 1920s, Etheldred Browning wrote about the housing problem and captured the predicament working women were facing: 'The word "home" generally conveys the idea of a husband as being attached, but because a woman supports herself and stands more or less alone, is this any reason that she must spend her days in a hostel or a bed-sitting room, and never arrive at the dignity of a home?'[44] Society has evolved since then, but I wonder how many of us still consider 'home' only as a place we share with a romantic partner.

Campaigns for equal pay intensified during the Second World War, when there was another huge influx of women into the workforce as the men were called up to serve. This increase in the proportion of women rose from 26 per cent (5.1 million) in 1939 to 36 per cent (just over 7.25 million) in 1943.[45] Newspaper articles from the time captured the urgent need there was for new, affordable housing that would cater for the growing number of single working women. There were some buildings designed for women living alone, such as the 50 flats in Waterlow Court in Hampstead Garden Suburb in north London, and Fiona House, a hostel for 70 women on Gray's Inn Road, also in London.[46] But women's pay remained, on average, just 53 per cent of the pay of the men they replaced,[47] and they were frequently refused mortgages if they didn't have the backing of male guarantors.

In 1964, women were allowed to share property equally with their husbands, thanks to the revision of the Married Woman's Property Act,[48] but a second wave of feminism really took off during the 1970s. The gains women made in that decade were a real breakthrough. In 1970, the Equal Pay Act made it illegal to discriminate against employees on the grounds of sex.

Women were legally able to get a mortgage of their own by 1995 when the Sex Discrimination Act forced banks to treat women and men equally. This came after a housebuilding boom, with 300,000 new homes built in England in 1955,[49] that peaked in 1968, when more than 425,000 new homes were completed.[50] Things looked to be improving but still, the numbers didn't add up. In 1976, the average house price in the UK ranged from £10,000 to £10,700,[51] while the average annual pay for women was £2,355 but £3,640 for men.[52] What's more, even though it was legal, banks were still refusing mortgages to women who didn't have a male guarantor into the late 1970s.[53]

However, women exercised their new-found freedom and, by 1981 in the USA, there were more single women homeowners (11 per cent of purchases) than single men homeowners (10 per cent).[54] This was the time that provided the inspiration for independent single women characters like Bridget Jones and Carrie Bradshaw; independent women who may have framed your understanding of what it means to 'live well' in your 30s. In the UK, the percentage of single women taking out a mortgage more than doubled, from 9.8 per cent in 1983 to 23 per cent in 2003.[55] When Margaret Thatcher was appointed as prime minister in 1979, 60 per cent of young adult women were in work. During the 1980s and 1990s, the gender pay gap slowly narrowed. In the USA, women's pay had increased from 64 per cent of men's in 1980 to 77 per cent by 2000.[56] The UK saw similar change, with women's average pay relative to men's increasing from 66 per cent in 1984 to 72 per cent in 2001.[57] In the UK in 1997, the average house price was just two-and-a-half times the average income for people in their mid to late 20s.[58]

One of Virginia Woolf's most famous works, *A Room of One's Own*, explores the position of women in society and the impact this has on the spaces they occupy. In 1929, Woolf wrote evocatively about the poverty of women, and how they could work and work, year after year, and still struggle to make ends meet.[59] In 2029, it will be a hundred years since *A Room of One's Own* was first published, yet many of the lines in it echo conversations I have with my female friends now. Women, despite the increase of their presence in the workplace, are still struggling to earn enough money to buy a home independently. It takes 5.3 years longer for a woman to save to buy a property in London than it does her male counterparts.[60] The only time I've been able to afford to rent independently, not in a house share, is when I moved in with a partner. One woman I interviewed for this book described the house share option as a 'waiting room' for women who want to own their own place and have yet to meet a partner to enable them to do so. Despite the outward advances that have been won for women in the workplace, in so many ways we have come full circle: unable to afford to buy our own place without cohabiting. If there's a silver lining to be seen in the fact that women before us experienced a similar thing, it's this: we can look to our predecessors' resourcefulness for guidance. In the 19th century, when the rising number of educated women in New England faced a similar problem, they chose to live together in partnerships that became known as a 'Boston marriage'.

Fun and fury

Realising that a conventional marriage at the time wouldn't allow them the space to pursue their intellectual and artistic goals, those entering into Boston marriages partnered with other women instead.[61] Some were romantically tied but others were purely platonic. Two women committed to living with each other so they could find the space to pursue a life they wanted outside the domestic sphere of marriage.

And here lies the flip side. Yes, women today are house sharing for longer than we'd like to. We might wish that we could afford a place of our own. We might be trying to meet a partner or our choices might be limited because of the gender pay gap. But something powerful happens when people – and, in my experience, women – come together to make 'a home for now' and help one another through the unique challenges of our generation.

When my life was in flux in my 20s, that house share with Phoebe, Sophie, and Jess was the only constant in my life for the three years I lived there. A few days before I turned 28, an Irish yoga teacher I'd been seeing for nine months, and who I'd fallen for, told me he didn't want to be in a relationship with me. He called to tell me this out of the blue while I was on my lunch break at work. I held it together at my desk for the last few hours of the working day, but when I got back to the kitchen that night and saw Phoebe and Sophie, it was them I confided in. It was my housemates who shared in my confusion, having witnessed the relationship unfold. They spent hours with me under a blanket on the sofa in our lounge, poring over the mixed signals and helping me to unpick a situation that I was struggling to understand. Their hugs and cups of tea were delivered with deep understanding, having endured painful dating scenarios themselves that year.

I was still processing the rejection – my first real encounter with heartbreak – when my 28th birthday arrived. I was rattling towards my 30s without the anchoring of the relationship I'd seen going somewhere or the type of home I thought I'd have by then. Then, at 2pm, my mum called for the second time that day. My grandad had died – my last remaining one.

It was my housemates who lifted me out of the hole I was in that day. Four garlic breads were baked in the Big Roasting Tin – a side dish to go with the gallon of spaghetti bolognese Jess was cooking. Phoebe finely grated a whole triangle of Parmesan. We extended the dining table with the desk from Sophie's room and plucked desk chairs and stools from all over the house so there was room for all of us, plus my sister, her husband, their two kids, and my best friend, Laura. They hung up a banner and readied a cake with candles. There I was, on my birthday, my Big Roasting Tin the centrepiece of a life so far from the one I'd imagined for myself – but a meaningful one.

It used to be that house sharing was a life stage sandwiched between other life stages, a transient place. But to reduce our house shares to being a waiting room of sorts is to deny ourselves ever feeling 'at home' in them. House shares are more than somewhere we can rest awhile until we get our lives together, they're a type of living situation to be celebrated in their own right. And when we allow ourselves to embrace that, we can invest in our homes – and ourselves.

2. Meeting Point

How to choose (good) housemates

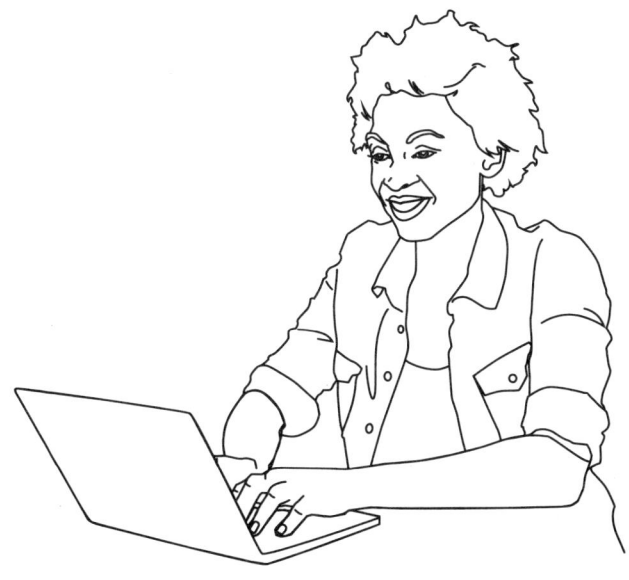

"When people show you who
they are, believe them"
Maya Angelou[1]

I'm perching on the edge of a third-hand bed that's been stripped down to the mattress, gathering strength to clean the filthy carpet under my feet – and to accept that this dingy, musty-smelling room that looks out on to the Old Kent Road in London is now home. I never met the room's previous occupier, but I'm in possession of his grubby sheets. I stash them in the wardrobe. It's SpareRoom – the equivalent of the lonely hearts pages for the unsettled – that brought me here, and this is my very first success story.

At this stage in my house sharing journey, I'm 23 and in that frantic, post-university haze, clawing back the independence I've had a taste of but unable to find a job to fund it. I'd spent too many weeks waking up in my childhood bedroom to commute two-and-a-half hours in to London, where I have an internship at a glossy magazine. Using the £50 a day they're paying me to rent a room in the city instead would bring me one step closer to adulthood. I just needed to find one I could afford within walking distance of my office.

I scrolled through the pages of SpareRoom's online catalogue and agonised over the messages I sent to unknown faces helpfully labelled by the platform as 'current flatmate'. If you've played the

SpareRoom game yourself, you'll know that it's surprisingly hard to sound like a normal human being, while also casually referencing that you're hygienic and law-abiding (but not neurotically so), laid back, but not *too* laid back. Someone they'd love hanging out with, but who has their own life. Signing off with times and dates I could view the room was the easy part.

I get a reply from 'Patrick'. This is good news because the room he was flogging in a house share of six (five others and, potentially, me) is cheap and a 20-minute walk from my office. In response to my rambling, subtly needy message, he writes:

'6 tonight works. At gym 6.30 tho.'

A 30-minute meeting usually means a light discussion. It's a time frame I associate with low-stakes life choices like a brief phone catch-up with my mum or a few laps round the park. In this one, I have to gauge if this could be my home and if the other five housemates are people I can see as my modern-day family of sorts.

There's a chaos to the Old Kent Road that, on dark winter evenings, is reduced to fast flashes of light – from buses, police cars, and blinking kebab shop signs. The disorder of the roundabout at its centre has a ripple effect on the streets around it. Walking them makes me hold my things tightly. I plug the road name in to Google Maps and let the arrow run inside my pocket, lifting my phone out every now and again to check I'm on track. I knock on the door and I'm met by a face that matches the one on SpareRoom. Patrick wordlessly ushers me inside. It's warm and I appreciate the vanilla Air Wick that's masking the smell of unwashed sportswear – a valiant attempt at domesticity that didn't require doing any actual washing.

I ask him if I can put the light on to see the room in its full glory and he pulls out his phone to switch his torch light on. Another workaround he'd thought of as all the light bulbs needed replacing. Patrick tells me that there are two others coming to view the room tomorrow. I weigh up my options: act now, take the room, and live as a fully functioning adult or risk losing it, continue the five-hour daily commute, and wake up staring at wallpaper I'd chosen when I was seven. In the low light of Patrick's phone torch, the room felt quite cosy. I'd make it work.

Maybe this would make a good meet cute in a film. Two unassuming souls cross paths in an unlikely spot and endure a few painfully tense minutes that leave us wondering, 'Will they? Won't they?' In films, usually they do and the rocky road to romance begins – and it's a road well travelled. Dissected and analysed by generations of experts, relationship psychotherapists and anthropologists, when I last checked, there were more than 60,000 books in Amazon's 'Dating' section, including *How to Get a Date Worth Keeping* and *The Grown Woman's Guide to Online Dating*. Each one pores over the details of that dance between two strangers deciding whether they're the right fit for each other. To the best of my knowledge, few of these meet cutes end with the two lovers, moments after meeting, moving in together, immediately sharing bills, meals, routines.

And yet, on multiple occasions, I have moved into a house share and, within hours, entrusted perfect strangers with my finances, happily conformed to their routines, and signed a contract legally binding myself to do so for the foreseeable future. You'll likely have done the same. Building such a level of intimacy at speed is something only housemates do, deciding to make the relationship a success after one meeting – and with a hefty deposit riding on it. Perhaps if, as with dating, we were more discerning and there was more of an open conversation about what we're looking for in a housemate, the house sharing journey would be a smoother one.

Intimacy on fast-forward

Now safely in my 30s, I know it's the people who create a sense of belonging for me, more so than the space. Being surrounded by people who are invested in me and considerate of my needs – as

I am of theirs – is what makes a place feel like home. Perhaps the search for good housemates and a good house share is actually like a search for a kind of surrogate family. A search for people who, for the time we live together, I will care about and will care about me. People who will accept and respect my quirks because I will do the same for them. Quirks like taking up space in communal areas with my creative projects or my strong aversion to wet bath mats left on the floor. Of the 2,000 British men and women surveyed by YouGov, 89 per cent said that they see their homes as a sanctuary where they can be themselves.[2] And young professionals working in today's 'always on' culture need somewhere to rest and restore as much as anyone. Surely it's the people you live with who have the power to create that.

The modern-day house share turns what we know about human bonding on its head. Living together is something that romantic couples and families can take years to truly master. When housemates do it after one meeting, it creates a somewhat unnatural connection. Perhaps you've felt it after moving in with strangers too. You very quickly know the intricacies of their shower routine and will be able to identify their clean socks on an airer by the scent of their washing powder, but not know their surname or where their office is. Some of us can spend more waking hours with our housemates than we do with our best friend, but still never feel close to them.

In 1993, the results of research by Professor Robin Dunbar, an anthropologist and evolutionary psychologist at the University of Oxford, were published and his conclusion has since become widely known as 'Dunbar's number'.[3] This is the number of people each individual can maintain stable and social relationships with, based on our cognitive limit as human beings. Robin's research suggests that we can maintain a maximum of only 150 meaningful human connections at once and these are highly structured. That total includes, at the centre, your circle of five closest, intimate relationships, then, in further concentric circles, 15 close friends, and then 50 friends outside that. The rest sit outside that, on the periphery.

I ask Robin for his insights on how the bonding psychology behind his research plays out in a house share set-up. 'Spending a lot of time with a housemate who you don't feel that close to does create confusion in our minds,' he says. 'If you think about being stuck in a lift with a stranger, we tend to go silent and stare at our feet. The physical closeness is not indicative of the closeness of the relationship. It's at odds. There are ways to engineer closeness through social activities, but you have to establish a baseline relationship before you can do that.'

Creating a relationship with someone we don't know relies on a number of psychological processes that kick in almost immediately after we meet them. It's these that influence our decisions about where in our social structure we want this person to sit and – more crucially when we're house share hunting – whether we want to live with them.

Consciously or not, our character and outlook on life weighs in on how we read a situation. In 2015, research on interpersonal chemistry[4] identified that participants who are agreeable, conscientious, female, and young are the most likely to report experiencing friendship chemistry. I'd say there's a high chance that these participants' agreeable and conscientious nature gets the better of them: they experience friendship chemistry because they want to feel it.

You're also more likely to make the effort to nurture a connection if you meet someone and perceive the relationship to be rewarding in some way, thanks to what psychologists call interdependence theory. That undoubtedly comes into play when you meet a housemate who can offer you a place to live and the less desirable alternative is to go back to searching on SpareRoom.

We also rely on 'notions of normalcy'. They're the conclusions we draw about people's personalities, based on previous experiences and reference points we have gathered from the people in our life. They influence how we perceive new people. In research in 2015, 2,000 participants took part in a platonic speed-dating exercise in which they had three minutes to get acquainted with a stranger and then assess their personality.[5] Based on their findings, researchers concluded that when we meet new people we tend to have a positive bias that leads us to assume they're just like the average person. When your mind is swaying you into thinking everyone you meet via SpareRoom is fine – near enough normal by your standards – the challenge you face is finding ways to make sure that really is the case. Ideally, before you sign the contract.

Chemistry or compatibility?

There's nothing like moving in with someone quickly, then realising it's not a good match, to make you hyper-aware that your first impressions can be unreliable. The truth is, the psychological processes at play when we meet a prospective housemate aren't all that trustworthy. In fact, they may even trip us up as our conscientious personality tricks us into thinking there's friendship chemistry when maybe there isn't or else we assume that someone has an average character only to find out, months later, they're actually very extreme in their views. And here lies the issue when it comes to making a decision about a housemate after only 30 minutes with them.

It takes time to build the foundations of a good relationship and to put our first impressions to the test. There's a reason why most of us spend months dating before making a romantic relationship official and why close friendships can often take years to build. There's a long information-gathering phase that helps to form this solid foundation. And yet, in a world where there are more housemates searching than there are rooms available, and there's financial pressure to fill a room so the rent gets paid, either way round we're forced to move quickly.

The house sharing scene we find ourselves in doesn't allow for an information-gathering phase. When fellow house sharers describe the confusion they feel when they're faced with complicated housemate relations, I have a strong suspicion that there's a bad housemate-matching process at the core of it. Perhaps you have a long list of your own house sharing nightmares and can map them back to a rash decision or an inaccurate first impression. The stories I hear from fellow house sharers about housemates who don't come out of their rooms, walk around with their earphones in, not wanting to engage in conversation, send passive-aggressive text messages, stop talking to them without a word as to why, have wild parties that keep everyone awake on weeknights… all began with a decision made quickly and out of necessity. There is often simply no time to put our compatibility to the test before committing to living with each other. No wonder so many of us find ourselves perplexed by the people we live with.

Eliza Moore, 36, has had her fair share of housemate disasters. She's a nanny from New Zealand and has lived in the UK for eight and a half years. She, too, says that the disasters could have been avoided by an improved housemate interview. She was living in a house in Brixton, London, when she and her friends desperately needed to find someone to fill a room. 'We scheduled 15-minute interviews for each person to come and have a drink with us. We went and bought a bunch of cans of cheap supermarket cider and offered them to everyone. So we were all getting progressively drunk and obviously, by the end of the night, the last guy that we saw is the guy we gave the room to. It was a big, big, big mistake because, obviously, this guy thought he had walked into the world's biggest party flat. There were so many red flags we missed: he was young and it was his first time living out of his parental home. He lost his keys a bunch of times. He would call my boyfriend at two in the morning being like, "I'm on my way home. Can you roll me a cigarette?" Just a nightmare. It was a horrible, horrible year.'

Years later, Eliza was looking to find another housemate to

take a room in that house share, this time in the middle of the Covid pandemic. 'It was so hard to fill the room because everyone was moving out of the city. There was only one guy interested. So we had to take him because we needed to pay the rent. He was so socially awkward. My friends and I ended up calling him an energy vampire. Basically, someone who will talk your ear off about the most mundane thing and just drain your will to live. I'm not exaggerating. If I ever got cornered in a conversation with him, I would lose an hour of my day. I'd find myself staying in my room until I heard him go back upstairs.'

Both Eliza's experiences highlight how the psychological processes we're relying on when we first meet someone aren't fit for purpose when it comes to choosing a good housemate in a short space of time. Her positive bias led to her making an assumption (albeit an alcohol-fuelled one in the first case) that the people they chose to fill the room in their house share would be fine. They were a nightmare. She chose the housemates because she had a problem to solve and they provided an answer. Maybe you've had to do the same. I know I have.

I let my need for a room cloud my decision when I first met Patrick. It's no wonder that, after his 10-minute tour of that Elephant and Castle house share, I only stayed in the room for six months. Patrick was a boozer and often woke me up on weeknights, bringing friends back and smoking weed outside my ground-floor window. When I first met him, I thought his predilection for Air Wick was a good sign, but I later realised he was heavily reliant on it to mask disgusting habits. He frequently washed his clothes without using detergent, and would let his friends sleep in my bed when I was away without telling me. I could always tell because my sheets smelled strongly of Davidoff Cool Water, and they'd leave telltale signs, like unfamiliar chargers in my plug sockets and used condoms tossed into my waste-paper bin.

So, after just six months, with the kind of desperate hope that spurs people to sign up to Tinder the same day that their relationship breaks down, I logged back on to SpareRoom. There were 18,202 London flat shares available, 1,939 in south east London alone. Accustomed to the high-resolution, full-width imagery of Airbnb, I looked through the tiny photographs of dark corners of spare rooms with suspicion. I'd get closer and closer to my laptop, looking for hidden clues as to what it might be like to live there. Is there a fruit bowl? Do they have loads of mismatched furniture? One flat I viewed had two dining tables crammed into the communal space and only two out of six chairs were safe to sit on. Good photography and interior design shine on this platform, so when I saw Emma's listing, I was already imagining myself washing up at her Belfast sink or curled up on her sofa. The flat overlooked a green, and there were high ceilings, natural light, and wooden floors lined with thriving plants. It was beautifully styled. She seemed like someone who would change the light bulbs.

The flat was in East Dulwich, a tree-lined part of south east London where there were more quirkily named cheesemongers than zebra crossings. Where the corner shops sell loose lentils and rice that you have to weigh out in paper bags. There's a park where you can take a pedalo out on the lake. Walking the streets of East Dulwich, the need to hold on to my things tightly felt less urgent than it had in Elephant and Castle.

I messaged 'current flatmate' Emma, editing the draft I'd originally sent to Patrick to tell her a bit about myself, and saying that I really liked the look of the flat. She, like me, worked in the creative industries and she grew up in rural Essex (I'm from rural Cambridgeshire). We seemed well matched.

I wanted to be more mindful this time about who I lived with, to make sure we connected in person. So, when I went round to view the flat, I stayed for a couple of beers. The conversation was polite but free-flowing. Emma had been there two years and spoke fondly of this time and the amenities surrounding the flat. She had been living with her boyfriend previously, but he was moving out to look after his mum, who was ill, so she needed another person to split the rent with. After I left, I got a text from her suggesting we meet for dinner the following week. A second date before we sealed the deal.

'Bonding is a long, slow process normally,' says Professor Robin Dunbar. 'But it can be fast-tracked by doing a number of social activities together that release endorphins: laughter, singing, dancing, feasting – so you could share a meal together. And storytelling – so sharing anecdotes and information about your life. These activities trigger the mechanism in our brain that underpins social bonding and creates a sense of closeness. We don't really know how long it takes. There's one study that looked at how long it takes to form a friendship and the figure was something like 200 hours over a period of months, which is only achievable if you don't have to work.'

It wasn't 200 hours' worth, but the amount of bonding time Emma was committing to was more than I was used to. The SpareRoom interactions I'd engaged in up to now had involved a bit of a preamble over the chat function before committing to a viewing time. I liked that Emma was taking it slow. We weren't rushing into this partnership of sorts. It needed to feel 'right'.

We met for dinner in a cosy pub on a street full of arty independent shops just across the green from Emma's flat. It was a warm evening after work in March and I felt all the anticipation of going on a date. She was there waiting with a couple of cold pints, remembering from our first meeting that it was my drink of choice.

It wasn't long before we were chatting away. Both the younger sisters of siblings with children, we bonded over our love of being aunties and shared photographs of our nieces. We talked about food – her chef boyfriend hosted supper clubs that she told me I should come along to. We compared our career journeys in our respective creative industries. They were similar. It had been tough, we agreed, but both of us felt as though we were over the mad hustle of poorly paid internships and working through the night.

We were two beers in when we decided we'd order some food. On second dates, that's a good sign. It was in this case, too, as the conversation was natural and neither of us wanted to leave. The sun shone through the pub window and I relaxed. I left elated at the prospect of a future in this high-ceilinged East Dulwich flat with my soon-to-be housemate who would welcome me into her ready-made supper-clubbing friendship group. It all sounded gloriously grown up. I never thought to ask questions that would confirm our compatibility.

Great expectations

There's an important distinction to be made between finding one or more housemates to live alongside who you get along with and actively seeking a housemate you want to be a friend. You might well hope to be friends with someone you move in with and make the necessary efforts to nurture a friendship. In my eyes, Emma and I had both shown willingness to put that effort in and were doing all the right things – things Robin would recommend we work on to create the foundations of our friendship. But, as with any relationship, you can't know how it will unfold.

'I think, in the end, the real issue with using a shortcut to build a bond, as you might when you're first meeting a prospective housemate, is that endorphin-based fuel for friendship might provide a platform for building a connection, but it won't make it last,' says Robin. 'The activities – the chemical tricks – they do seem to work for a while, but then it will come down to how much you have in common.'

At the very least, I felt sure that we had enough in common to be housemates. I was sure we could be good friends. So, when she offered me the room, I was thrilled that she clearly felt the same – we'd have a nice life living side by side in her beautiful East Dulwich flat. I signed on the dotted line, we set a date, and exchanged a few texts in the run-up to my moving in that sounded very much like two mature young women ready to share a home.

'Hey, Alice, hope you're getting excited for the move! Wondered if you want any of the furniture left in the room? Will get Chris to store if not. Ex'

'That's really kind but I'm all good – have just ordered a bed to get delivered the day I arrive x'

'Great! Do you need a hand on moving in day? x'

'Hi! Think I'll be OK. Not too much stuff. Do you have a French press there? I'll bring mine if not x'

Moving in day was a bright Saturday in April. I popped up to the second-floor flat luggage-free to announce my arrival before I started bringing in boxes. I thought maybe we'd have coffee and a catch-up before I started unloading. But I met Emma coming down the narrow stairwell. Hair up, sunglasses on, tote bag on shoulder. She was heading out. She was looking at the floor and hadn't taken her sunglasses off, so I asked if she was all right. Her boyfriend had ended things, she said, and she was going to get coffee with a friend to give me some space to move in. I responded as empathetically as I could, this being only the third time we'd met.

There was an atmosphere in the flat from the moment she returned. I couldn't shake the feeling that I was in her space. Spring passed and, in between being in the office and weekend plans, we'd touch base in the lounge every now and then, shuffling around each other in the flat. She'd have mates over who'd sit in the lounge with her and watch films, but she'd never introduce me. Then, when they'd gone, she'd shut herself in her room and I could hear her chatting on the phone for hours. I said a couple of times that I was there to listen if she needed to chat, cry, or drink wine. I wondered if the break-up was the reason I was getting this frosty side of her.

To draw her out of her room, I suggested we host some drinks at the flat for both our friends as a housewarming. All week we exchanged messages about the punch we were going to make and what day we were both free to go to the shop together to get supplies. Then, the night before, she told me that she and her friends were going out to a rave instead.

They assembled at our flat ahead of the rave to share a bag of housewarming coke that her friend, who called himself Sparrow, gifted her. I watched them sniff it off the *ELLE* magazine I hadn't finished reading yet. It was 4am when she rolled in that night. I know because, although I'd been asleep for an hour by then, I woke up to her having sex on the landing, against the wall of my room. I lay there, paralysed. Nothing in my life had prepared me with the tools I needed to escape from this awkward trap I was now stuck in. When Patrick used to wake me up, I'd open the door to my room and tell him to be quiet. If I opened my door to protest now, I'd see Emma and her late-night friend, naked, having sex. Ear plugs only blocked out the sex sounds to a certain extent as they were all the more uninhibited because Emma and friend were very high. I fell asleep at some point after a panicked text exchange with my sister Emily, who'd also been awake at 4am, nursing her toddler. She'd agreed, Emma's behaviour was out of order, but we settled on the explanation that it was probably a rebound thing and a one-off.

The next morning arrived and I made my way to the kitchen to start clearing up the bottles and glasses from the night before. I spritzed my *ELLE* magazine, front and back, with disinfectant. Emma walked in to make her visitor a coffee. I was expecting an acknowledgement at the very least, if not an apology. She didn't lift her gaze from the worktop to chat to me.

'Hey,' I said when she walked in.

'Ugh I feel like death,' she replied.

A short exchange followed, our awkward silences punctuated by the sound of me washing up and the clink of the teaspoon as she poured and stirred milk into their coffees. She started walking out of the kitchen, mugs in hand, and said, 'We're gonna order food.' She shut the door to her room, I later heard her leave to collect the food and I didn't see her again until Tuesday evening.

During the weeks that followed, I came to the stark realisation that Emma and I were not compatible as housemates after all. Maybe it was unfortunate that I was getting to know her in the middle of a break-up. Maybe she was more of a partier than me. Maybe she just didn't want for us to hang out together. I'll never know. But there were sleepless nights for me as multiple Tinder dates for her led to boozy parties for two in the living space that sat between our bedrooms. Even her ex came round to revisit their favourite sex spots one Wednesday night.

On the Thursday, after being kept up all night, I had to call in sick. I was freelancing then so I lost out on my day rate. The fact that I'd lost money gave me the kick I needed to bring it up with her. I sent her a long text because I couldn't face talking about her sex habits in person. I apologised for having to mention it but said I'd felt uncomfortable with the loud sex and that she needed to remember I was paying to live there too now. She apologised and did seem quite mortified. But, even with an apology, I didn't want to live with someone who was so unaware of the impact her behaviour had on me. I decided it was time to move on. By then, I had spent three months trying to navigate our differences. I couldn't understand how it had all gone so wrong. I'd done my due diligence – or, at least, I thought I had.

Finding good enough

I think I fell into all the mind traps possible when I met Emma. Looking back, it's easy to see the point at which your need to find a home clouded your decision making. I was relying on the relationship working out because I desperately needed to move out of my flat with Patrick, and fast. I had a vision and I needed her to like me to bring it to life. I took the few commonalities we had and assumed that she was just like me and had a similar lifestyle to mine. In my excitement at finding her East Dulwich flat and first meeting Emma, I'd made the mistake of forgetting to ask her some fundamental questions and putting my assumptions to the test.

As someone who is both generally conscientious and agreeable, I'd held back from sharing some of my own non-negotiables in case it rocked the boat. I hadn't thought that, unlike other relationships – romantic and friendship – this wasn't about me being likeable or even lovable, but was, first and foremost, about being compatible when living together. This, I think, is similar to what happens when you're dating someone and you feel a closeness – in part fuelled by sex as well as the endorphin-releasing activities that Robin identifies – and that feeling overrides your clear judgement when you're assessing the person in front of you. The connection and the feeling I got about Emma and living in the flat clouded the enquiring part of my brain. I never asked Emma how often she went on nights out, when she cleaned the flat, what time she went to bed, how often she saw her friends, what her work schedule was like, if she hoped to socialise with me, if she was into drugs, what her weekends looked like. I should have.

I think about Eliza, the nanny who lived in Brixton, and her journey alongside my own. I can see how, similar to dating in romantic relationships, we took what we learned from our bad house shares and used it to inform our decisions from then on to move forwards. By finding out what doesn't work for you, you're also getting a clearer idea what does.

'It is a long, slow process to get it right,' says Robin. 'My sense is that house shares can provide a stable base from which you might build a network of friends or community over time. My take on it would be that, at the very least, your house share provides you with an anchoring from which to develop your own interests and social life. If it all breaks up after a year or two, you've hopefully had enough time to build a wider community. If it works and creates lifelong friends, then it's not to be sniffed at.'

The housemate interview process is a crucial opportunity to learn about someone in a short space of time and to disclose what you're looking for from a housemate and a house share. It's important to get a sense of whether there's a connection there but, arguably, it's more important to glean the information you need to know to see whether you're compatible.

I struggled with accepting that it was OK and perfectly normal for a housemate not to become a friend. Like most of us, I'd grown up around schoolfriends and lived with people at university who became friends. So when I moved into a professional house share, it was the first time I was encountering this new type of relationship: not a friend but more than an acquaintance. I think there's a need to normalise and unpack this sort of less intense type of housemate relationship – one that doesn't sit within the structures we're familiar with.

I see now how building a less intense housemate relationship that remains steady is a beneficial approach. There's a real need to celebrate housemate relationships that are simply good enough – where you rub along just fine, your values align far enough for you to live together amicably, and you care about one another to a certain extent, but they remain less intense, low-stakes relationships.

'Weak ties' is what Dr Meg Jay,[6] a clinical psychologist and author, calls these low-stakes connections. She advocates looking outside our 'urban tribes' and suggests that living with close, like-minded friends in your inner circle can actually limit your personal and professional growth, whereas someone on the periphery of your circle could present opportunities. 'Weak ties promote, and sometimes even force, thoughtful growth and change,' she says.

Eliza, the nanny who mistakenly gave the impression her

Brixton home was a party flat, has moved twice since then. Now she, like plenty of women I speak to, actively chooses not to live with friends and enjoys the set-up she's currently in where they are friendly towards one another but don't socialise together. She's refined what she needs from a housemate: someone with some social skills, who can hold a conversation, and who doesn't clash with her values.

It's not that Eliza doesn't care who she lives with, but there are certain criteria she focuses on. As she puts it, 'Everyone wants to get along with the people they live with. No one wants a toxic home environment, but my bar is very low. I want to get along with my housemates and I'll stand in the kitchen and chat to them for ages, but now I'm older and I have my social circle, I don't have the time or energy to invest in socialising with my housemates. I'm not saying I'm going to move in somewhere and act like an asshole, but this is where I sleep and keep my clothes and that's it. From the general vibe of both the ad I responded to and the meet-up with them, it was clear that it would be great if we all got along but we've got our own stuff going on.'

When a room in her current house share became available, the remaining housemates decided to cover the rent for a month rather than rush to fill the room with someone who wasn't a good fit. So there's still a selection process when you're living with weak ties, and it's still a good idea to give it time and thought to make sure it's a good match.

Pausing like this to make room for an information-gathering phase before moving in to a house share or choosing a housemate isn't something that comes naturally when we're under pressure to find somewhere to live. I know that, whenever I've been looking, the need to find a place to live has always felt very immediate because I wasn't happy where I was living, I was starting a new job, or I'd given notice on an existing contract. I've always felt under time and financial pressure to find somewhere, which makes it hard to hold out for the right person.

I've learned to see it as a kindness to myself to give the searching process the time and head space it warrants, even when that doesn't feel very practical. Lodging in a friend's spare room, sofa surfing, and staying with my mum for stints in between house shares meant I didn't need to rush into signing myself up to a contract I was unsure about.

I entered my eighth house share last year at the age of 32: a new-build two-bed flat in Bow in London that overlooks the canal. The excitement I felt about going to live there reminded me of how I'd felt about Emma's East Dulwich flat. I'd recently broken up with my boyfriend and this flat represented a new beginning. I wanted to live there so badly – imagining myself in this new area, which was close to my friends and an easy commute to work – but this time, equipped with all I'd learned, I remembered to keep my feet on the ground.

I met Martha, my new prospective housemate, with my eyes wide open. I had my list of non-negotiables and I'd viewed a few other flats already, so they rolled off my tongue very easily when we met for my first viewing. I had to keep reminding myself that this process wasn't about being liked. I viewed the room and asked lots of practical questions about the place. And then, over a cup of tea, I bit the bullet and asked her what her dating habits were, whether she went out a lot, how her relationship with her last housemate had been, how she spent her weekends, and if she hoped we would hang out together occasionally.

Having prepared these questions in my mind ahead of time made it a lot easier to focus on compatibility and not get swept up in the connection I was feeling. I did really like her as a person and we bonded over each other's funny dating and work stories, but I was able to put the laughter and likeability factors to one side during the interview. I reminded myself that these might be a sign of a connection, but they're not the sign of a good housemate, so I still needed to dig deeper to get to the practicalities, which would make our house share a happy place – or not.

I opened up about my house share with Emma and how I'd learned that I couldn't live with a partier, and she shared with me her own concerns about living with someone who might regularly bring unfamiliar men back to the flat and disrupt the calm. Also that she had a dog visit sometimes. I told her that I'm not a massive dog person but I quite like walking them. Opening this honest conversation revealed a lot about her, and me, and I could see that we had similar ideas about how we would live together. It is, to date, the best house share I have lived in: one defined by mutual respect, shared values (or enough of them), and realistic expectations. I put this down to the fact that, by asking myself the questions in the next section, I was able to take the time to reflect and iron out what was going to work and not work for me in a house share and what I was looking for in a housemate.

Chapter reflections
What are your non-negotiables in a house share?
Approach the information-gathering phase by first making a list of your non-negotiables. Maybe it's that you want your partner to stay twice a week or you love cooking and want to make it clear from the beginning that you will be in the kitchen a lot. Ask others who have lived with you for information that they think might be important for your future housemates and reflect on past experiences of what you've liked or not liked in previous housemates. The more you can share up front, the better. It's important to remember to stop yourself getting caught up in being liked: this is about finding housemates who are compatible with how you want to live.

What do the people who know you well think about the house share and the housemates you're considering moving in with?
Taking time to discuss prospective housemates and house shares with the people who know me best was really valuable. Sometimes they pointed things out that I hadn't thought of or I'd mentioned were a priority and helped me to hold out for the right thing when I was tempted to accept something that wasn't quite right.

What does your ideal house share look like?

When you think about your dream house share, are you living with friends or people who feel familiar but aren't too involved in your life? How many? How often do you see one another? What agreements or parameters are in place? Is there a good balance between having your own space and the option to chat in communal spaces? Whether you're imagining a big kitchen where you all sit and eat together of an evening or a peaceful space where you can enjoy solitude, write down or draw a mind map of all the things that are important to you in a house share scenario. Keep this image in mind when you are searching or perhaps think about how you might adapt your current situation so it aligns more closely with this vision.

What are your red and green flags for housemates?

Make a list. It's taken me seven house shares to get a clear picture of what these flags are so feel free to use mine as a starting point, changing or adding more of your own that come to mind.

Red flags
- Looking for a temporary living fix.
- Not committed to making the house share feel like home.
- Bad work–life balance.
- Party animal (excessive drink and drugs).
- Brash or very loud.

Green flags
- Positive anecdotes of previous house shares.
- Clear idea of what they're looking for (ideally, for the house to feel like home).
- Balance of social activities and relaxation.
- Considerate.

What are your ideal policies for a house share?

Write a short sentence stating what your ideal policy is for each of the following aspects of living together so you have it clear in your mind what you're looking for when you discuss them with your potential housemates. I have given an example in each case to help get you started.

- **Having guests over** Friends and family are welcome, but it would be good to float the dates and arrangements in the group chat before commiting to them.
- **Having partners over** Partners are welcome so long as the balance works for all the housemates.
- **Sex** Only in the bedrooms.
- **Bills** If someone's late with payment, there needs to be a chat and a commitment about a better way to handle this.
- **Cleaning** There'll be a rota for the kitchen and bathroom. Bedrooms are down to the individual.
- **Working from home** Up to three days a week is fine. If it stretches to five, there'll need to be a discussion about arrangements for heating during the winter. Laptops shouldn't be in communal spaces in the evenings or at weekends.

Write your list of proposed policies out and share it with your house. WhatsApp it to your housemates for them to comment on. Having one sentence for each aspect that everyone agrees with is an informal way of getting their buy-in and gauging people's thoughts. You can also share it when looking for new housemates, saying, 'Hey, I'm reading this book and it advises that, in a house share, we have an outline policy on having guests over, having partners over, sex, bills, and cleaning. I've written this. Do you feel like that's how we approach things? It'd be great to shape this together...'

3. Peas in a Pod

How to navigate living with friends

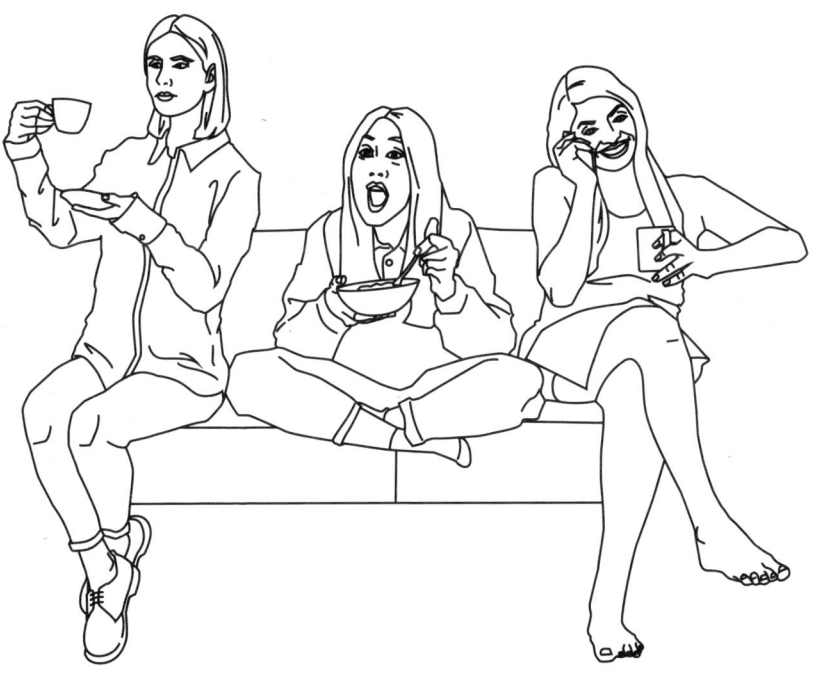

"True friendship is about taking it easy on each other, knowing
that life has tides that take you to various places, and that
you'll find a way back to each other at different points"
Dolly Alderton[1]

If you own an iPhone, you'll know how it likes to curate your
photos into 'on this day' videos and organise them into categories
like 'by the coast' and 'furry friends'. You'll also be familiar with
how, in the 'people' section, it catalogues faces that it's identified
as being significant to you. Mine is a visual record of all the
housemates I've lived with over the years.

It's a line-up of all the kinds of friendships I've experienced
living in house shares: old, new, fleeting, long-term, and everything
in between. These faces were – as my iPhone correctly identified
– intensely involved in my life. Now, they elicit a range of feelings
based on how the time we lived together went.

Some of the faces, it takes me a moment to place. Like Ally. I
lived with her for six months and, when I flick through photos of
a holiday we went on to Lake Garda – her in summer dresses and
sunglasses posing in doorways or sipping wine – I smile,
remembering how, in the short time we lived together, we'd share
clothes and be each other's plus ones to work socials. We lost
touch when she moved out and I haven't spoken to her since.

On other days, there are photos of the year I spent with Sima and Lottie. Snaps of the summer we hosted a barbeque in our gravel-surfaced front garden that looked on to a bus stop. The Halloween house party when we built a scarecrow. All of us in neon-orange life jackets on a stormy boat trip we took in Amsterdam. I'll forward those ones immediately to our 'Three Women' WhatsApp group for us to reminisce because, despite all having moved house at least four times in the 10 years since we house shared, we are still good friends.

When 'on this day' photos appear of the three years I lived with my school friend of 10 years, Phoebe, I'm awash with a mixture of complicated feelings. Photos of sharing fish and chips suppers in the park by our flat after work and going for post-dinner strolls to the ice cream shop on the corner of our road are tinged with memories of the difficult times we shared while living together. I really believed that I knew how to be a good friend and maintain a friendship, until I moved into a house share with this friend.

What makes friendship so wonderful is that, by its very nature, it is optional and entirely your choice. There's a breeziness that comes with that. It's what makes it so special when friends show up. They don't have to, but they choose to. This very quality is what makes friendship so light and free; it also makes it fragile.

In my house shares – and perhaps you've observed the same in yours – the friendships are high up in the hierarchy of types of relationships people have. Perhaps because the people living in my house shares have been either single or chosen not to live with a partner, friendships naturally occupied a big space in their lives – and in mine. Putting friendships top seems to be part of a generational shift, with 55 per cent of 16–39-year-olds in the USA saying that friendship is more important to them than a romantic relationship.[2] We invest time, energy, and emotion in our friendships, and with that investment comes hope, expectation, and an element of risk.

I know how special it can be living with a friend. I also know only too well the off-the-scale state of precariousness that can come from living with a friend. To stay sane and live happily with a friend in a house share, we must strike a careful balance between the highs and lows, intensity and distance, support and disappointment.

The sky's the limit, but a house share has four walls

After 10 years of friendship, I decided to move into the house share my school friend Phoebe had been living in for a year already. Knowing how well we got on, the prospect of living together was exciting. We'd met in sixth form, when both of us had dramatic side fringes and wore tank tops as skirts. Then, here we were, years later, with better hair, living in next-door rooms in a flat in Balham, London. At 16, we'd bonded over our similar tastes in books and art and a love of drinking tea while overanalysing our lives. A decade later – in a different city and in actual jobs – we went to book talks and art exhibitions together, met at fancy wine bars and continued to drink tea and anaylse life.

I ask Professor Robin Dunbar, an anthropologist and evolutionary psychologist at the University of Oxford, for his insights on friendship in house shares. You might remember, I mentioned his research into friendship in Chapter 2 and how his conclusion that 150 is the number of people you can maintain stable and social relationships with has become widely known as 'Dunbar's number'.[3] Drawing on his own and others' research in this field, he made some interesting observations.

'It's important to note that the dynamics of bonding in friendships tend to be very different between the two sexes,' he says. 'Social psychologists have done a lot of research on this. So, women's relationships are generally much more one on one and focused compared with men's bonding style, which is usually very casual and based on convenience. It means that, often, female friendships can be more intense and, as a result, a more fragile form of friendship. Because female friendships tend to be closer, there's more opportunity for them to fracture and fracture terminally, so there is a risk involved here. The question is, how do you negotiate that while living together?' Between the importance placed on friendship because of the life stage most house sharers are in and the fragility of female friendship, living with a friend in a house share presents an obstacle course of joyful moments and potential pitfalls.

I'm in my mid-20s in this house share and Phoebe spans both ends of my life so far, which is rare: she knows my family and where I grew up *and* she knows the names of my colleagues and friends in London. I feel whole talking to her. Whenever I arrive back at the flat after visiting my family, she wants to hear how everyone is – and not just a polite ask, she wants a proper conversation, to see photographs, and displays genuine interest. I want to hear the same level of update, too, when she returns from her family home. I know her boyfriend, Ben, who has become part of our friendship group during their three years together. When he visits and our other two housemates are out, he'll cook and the three of us eat together, operating like a functional extended family.

My room here, tucked away on the third floor of the Victorian terrace in Balham, is the warmest room in the flat. So toasty that sometimes, even in the colder months, I crack open the door to the Juliet balcony to let in some of the icy air. I'm used to keeping warm in house shares by relying on electric blankets and wearing hats to bed, so this is luxury. On winter mornings, I draw back the curtains and watch the light projecting on to the walls opposite. Sometimes I'll go downstairs to make a tea and return to that very spot to revel in the tranquillity, a joy savoured after the chaos of the house shares that had come before this one. It's not lost on me how much of this being-at-home feeling comes from knowing that one of my oldest, closest friends is just across the landing.

As a house, parkruns are our thing. I wake up on Saturday mornings to hear the others getting their running gear on and know how my morning will unfold. We'll find one another after our run, get coffee, return home rosy cheeked, make breakfast, chat in front of *Saturday Kitchen*, and take it in turns to shower.

It's six months into my time living aboard the smooth-sailing house share when a text in the house chat rocks the boat. Before I moved in, Phoebe confided in me that she was having problems with some of her housemates being difficult about how often Ben was staying over. When we were chatting about me moving in, I asked her how often she was seeing Ben – an attempt to be up front so it wouldn't cause us issues down the line. She'd said three nights a week, but some of those she'd go to his. Now that I'm here, I'm noticing that Ben is staying in our flat every evening and then during the day when we're at work. A couple of days ago, there was a very awkward encounter when I was working from home – a rare occurrence – and, at 2pm in the afternoon, he let himself in with a key I didn't know he had to drop off a bag. He was as shocked to see me as I was to see him.

I look back on it today, five years later, and think Phoebe and I got a lot right when we lived together. We dedicated time to just us as a pair, we respected that there were some evenings when we wanted to be alone, and we also operated as a team in the wider group. Without realising it, we were working at maintaining our existing relationship as well as giving ourselves, and the friendship, room to grow. But there was also a lot we got wrong.

Now, I listen intently and with invested interest to others who are going through difficult times with friends. Often, they remedy it by taking a bit of time away from one another. That is not an easy option in a house share, where you are contractually obliged to share living quarters.

When you introduce the confines of a physical space, the relationships shift. As Professor Ho Law, who specialises in coaching and mentoring psychology, points out, there are parallels to be drawn between the transition a friendship goes through when it moves from being friends who socialise to friends who cohabit and the transition romantic partners experience when they move in together.

'As a psychologist, I believe the sky's the limit and so is the mind, but a house is a physical space and so it's limited, and living in it requires a lot of compromise. Your behaviour is always going to directly impact the other person who is present in the space. At the most basic level, there will be times that both of you need to go to the bathroom. The physical space adds a whole other layer to a romantic relationship and a friendship in a house share.

'There are multiple factors at play. You have the financial, the practical, and then also the emotional. You project what you hope living with that person will be like, but you don't have the whole picture until you've lived with that person day in, day out. And, just like when romantic partners cohabit, there's a tension between the heart and mind.'

Conscious cohabiting

Getting to know someone better means seeing the different sides and new depths of their personality. There's a stage that psychologists observe in the development of romantic couples' relationships called 'differentiation'.[4] In biology, differentiation is a process whereby cells evolve to become specialised. In a relationship, it's a process that occurs after a couple has become established and each person begins carving out space for their individual thoughts and personality within the relationship – their differences. I also see this happening with friends who move in to house shares and become housemates.

The differentiation phase can feel disappointing – peppered with conflict as imperfections come to light. There's a realisation that there are parts of each other you don't like and beliefs you don't agree with.

If partners conquer this stage, they enter what author and relationship awareness therapist Dr Alexandra H. Solomon calls 'brave love'.[5] Rather than avoiding the differences or them being too big for them to live with, they find healthy ways to live alongside them and handle conflicts. She pinpoints brave love as being a good point to move in with a partner, as then there are coping mechanisms in place to resolve differences.

But friends moving in to a house share have likely never reached that differentiation stage, when they're comfortable pointing out their differences and dealing with conflicts that might arise as a result. I certainly hadn't before I moved in with Phoebe. And without this accepted structure to the progression of a romantic relationship – where we might have been more likely to discuss our future, spend more time together in a close domestic space to test out our compatibility, and have more of a discussion about how living together would unfold – friends who move in together are left to see what happens, to find out if our differences will make or break us.

There's a clear distinction between couples who make an intentional choice to move in together and others who just fall into it according to researchers at the Center for Marital and Family Studies at the University of Denver.[6] Their work on 'sliding versus deciding' in relation to cohabiting makes a case for it being better for couples to decide to do so, not slide into it. They observed that a lack of awareness in the decision-making phase is often reflected in the cohabiting stage, with couples who slide being less proactive in terms of doing things to help the relationship thrive.

Friends can often 'slide' into living with each other, too – not putting the same weight on the importance of the preparation needed when moving in with a friend that we might with a romantic partner. It's deemed a casual move, often taken lightly. But, as Ho points out, it is still a big step that carries emotional risk for you and the friendship. 'You have to remember that there's an emotional engagement and an investment beyond the financial,' he says. 'You emotionally invest in that friendship and housemate. And with that, there's a rising risk of rejection. The more you invest, the more significant the loss will be. Living together is a big shift and the adjustment will take time and effort.'

If, before living together, while the stakes are low, we can be more aligned in terms of what we want out of our friendship while living together, this would help to iron out any discrepancies in our expectations of each other. It's trickier, though not impossible, to retrofit something like this after you've lived together for a while. Think about things that have caused friction in your friendships before and how, in a best-case scenario, you'd like to remedy those things with your friend in your house share. It might be that you know you'd like to socialise separately from the friend when you're living with them, seeing mutual friends alone sometimes, and you'd like your friend to understand that it's not personal, just something you'd like to keep separate. It might be that you'd like to be able to date without your friend enquiring about it or sharing their opinion. Think of it like a psychological contract of sorts.

While cohabiting romantic partners are more likely to be committed to each other, planning a future together and having conversations to scope what that will look like, friends living together in a house share know it'll be a temporary measure. 'In lifelong relationships like marriage or romantic partnerships, there's a lot of compromise, but in a house share, even if you're friends, people are less inclined to make compromises or they aren't explicitly discussed because the relationship isn't lifelong, so people see less benefit from that investment,' explains Ho. 'Whether you're aware of it or not, we tend to do a sort of cost and benefit analysis. We weigh up the pros and cons of what we're putting in and what we're getting out of our relationships. What we gain determines what we give back.'

It makes sense that, in a house share where you envisage living for only a few years, you might avoid facing up to your differences with a friend or compromising too much just so you can live together side by side conflict-free. You're certainly not going to compromise on something that means a lot to you for a house share if you'll only be living there for a short time.

Tipping point

Nonetheless, the level of compromise required when you're sharing a physical space challenges the breeziness that makes most friendships – and, indeed, fledging romantic relationships – thrive. But, as you'll know, there are some compromises you make for housemates that are easier to swallow than others. Waiting to use the bathroom because your housemate is in the shower is one thing. But waiting to use the bathroom when Phoebe and Ben were camping out in there for two hours, taking books and snacks in with them, was another. As far as I could tell, she was in the bath and he was sitting on the toilet chatting to her, and then they'd swap and he'd wash while she sat and chatted to him. Fine, if there wasn't a queue of three other housemates waiting for the facilities.

Then came The Text.

JESS: Anyone borrowed some kitty money? There was £45 in the jar and now only £5 x

PHOEBE: I haven't xxxx

ME: I haven't either x

SOPHIE: Nor me… x

That evening, home from work, it was only Jess and me.

'Bit worrying about the money. Has it happened before?' I asked her outright.

'Yeah, it's so random. Like, it's fine for a few months and then stuff will just disappear. And we think we've noticed some alcohol going missing, too. I had a whole bottle of vodka and now it's just empty. And some wine went missing. But it's so random and sporadic, it's kind of hard to know if it's my imagination. But the money, for sure, there was £45 and now only £5.'

'God. And it's not like any of us drink loads or don't have money. Like, if I'd polished off a bottle of vodka, you'd know about it.'

'Yeah.' Jess looked me. Without saying anything, I think we both had the same suspicion. The only person other than us four was Phoebe's boyfriend, Ben.

As more money and alcohol went missing, sometimes from our bedrooms, the tension in the house was reaching new levels. Sophie, feeling anxious and unsafe, moved out for a couple of weeks to live with her mum. I tried gently suggesting to Phoebe that Ben didn't stay in the house when we weren't in – to alleviate any suspicions that it may be him stealing from us. But he continued to be round all the time.

Then, I found a bottle of gin stashed in the cistern of the toilet. When I noticed Ben visiting the bathroom more than was natural, it confirmed my suspicions that it was him who had been stealing our alcohol and our money.

To date, it's the hardest conversation I have had to have. In a café in Balham on a dark winter's evening, I had to find the right words to tell one of my oldest friends that I thought her partner had a drinking problem and he was stealing from us.

It's not how I imagined living together would go. We thought it would simply be an extension of how wonderful our friendship had been so far. We were so excited. But neither of us had prepared for this new dynamic in which her partner's problems were now also my problems, and my anxieties were also her anxieties. Until this point in our friendship, we'd maintained a line. Our respective emotional baggage was kept mostly to ourselves, with the occasional opening up and sharing of things that you do with friends. Living together, that line wasn't just blurry, it was non-existent.

Ben terrorised our flat after that, turning up drunk and bashing on the door multiple times until, finally, I called the police. Back then, I didn't have the knowledge, understanding. or tools to know the best way to deal with the dramatic and uncomfortable overlap of these two worlds, where what was happening in my friendship was disrupting my home. Aware of how much pain Phoebe was in as she was trying to unpick her relationship, I managed my own feelings as best I could. But I was so unsettled and disturbed by Ben and his behaviour, I arrived at work one morning in tears, so I went to live with my mum for a couple of weeks.

I never spoke to Phoebe about how distressed I was. It never felt appropriate when she had her own, very urgent, emotions to work through. Now, as a 33-year-old woman, with more awareness of how enveloping coercive relationships can be, I have more empathy and understanding available for Phoebe than I could muster then. At the time, not knowing what to do, I was angry about how she'd let him into our safe space, how unsettled he made me feel, how much of an impact it had on everyone else in the house – and for so long. I continued to find bottles of alcohol stashed in hiding places around the flat, but I didn't tell her, not wanting to make the situation worse.

Breaking the fourth wall of friendship

As friends who live together, you see all parts of your friends' lives – parts that they may not want you to see and you might never have been party to if you weren't living together. Usually, you can choose what you share with your friends and when. When you're living together, you can't, and it shakes the foundations of the friendship – a relationship that, for the most part, works because you celebrate the things you have in common.

Hannah Mitchell, 40, works in PR and now lives in Norwich, following a nine-year stint of living in house shares with other professionals in London. For the first few years she was house sharing, she lived with a close friend – someone she'd known for 15 years – in house shares with two or three other housemates besides them. As in my case, living together presented challenges for their friendship.

'Before we lived together, I'd see her three times a year at least to go on holiday or to festivals, or we'd just visit each other. It was exciting when she initially moved in, but issues cropped up within a few months of living together. We had disagreements about bad habits in the house. Her approach to dating and relationships was disruptive for the house as she'd often have people over all the time. She just didn't seem to understand that her behaviour had an impact on others. By the time we'd lived together for three years, we were making less effort with each other. Whenever we did hang out, we'd end up talking loads about stuff happening in the house. We had mutual friends but sometimes – to escape all that was going on in the house – I just wanted to have a night out with someone else, someone independent from the house, and talk about other things. So there were times when I'd do things with our mutual friends separately, which started to cause a bit of friction.

'No matter how good friends you are, living with each other is intense. When I think back to the things that caused friction, they seem really trivial. But when you're living together, these things magnify. In the end, she decided to move out to protect our friendship. We had a calm and measured conversation about it and, as soon as she'd moved out, we went back to dedicating time to each other. Simply not living together improved everything and we're still great friends.'

Both Hannah and I, in living with our school friends, took the friendship out of the context in which it was formed, prising it from the roots that had anchored it. Our friendships made sense when we met at school and then when we'd choose to catch up doing fun things in the years that followed. We tag our friends according to where we met them: work friends, home friends, university friends, school friends, gym friends.

By living with each other, you're asking that connection to withstand a whole new, more intense dimension. In an article on friendship in *The Atlantic*,[7] Emily Langan, a communication professor and close relationship researcher, talks about how the context shifts in friendships when you try keeping in touch with friends you've made in real life via social media. 'It violates what I'll call the camp-friend rule of commemorative friendship. No matter how close you were with your best friend from summer camp, it is always awkward to try to stay in touch when school starts again. Because your camp self is not your school self, and it dilutes the magic of the memory a little to try to attempt a pale imitation of what you had.'

Perhaps the same is true of living with a friend in a house share. In my case, the school friend self is not the housemate self. I think it's why, in my experience, new friendships that have been formed in house shares tend to survive because, then, they are based on the self you are when you are living together. You decide on the ties you want to make and how tightly you want them to be knotted. It's low risk compared with living with an established friend you've known for years.

The honesty policy

Hayley Freeman, 31, who works in communications for a charity and lived with her friend Rachel from school for three years, says that she wouldn't have done it any other way. Still, she pinpoints how it was external influences that caused the most friction when they lived together.

'It was like the two of us were in a sort of relationship ourselves. Whenever I was single, it would be Rachel I spent my Saturday night with, but then I'd be dating and meet someone and it would be like trading one person in for the other and it felt really harsh. She'd do the same thing to me and it was awful to be on that side of things – you just felt like you had no one while the other one was loved up.

'We had different goals, too, because even when Rachel was with a boyfriend, she couldn't afford to rent as a couple, so always wanted to rent as a three with me. But I wanted to meet someone and move in with them because I could afford to rent a place to ourselves. Actually, after a year living together, I was about to move out with a boyfriend when I discovered – on the day we were moving – that he was cheating on me. I was obviously distraught, and I needed Rachel to be kind enough to make a U-turn and stay living with me, which she did.

'By the second year, we'd settled into living together. We even started sharing my car and had this sort of picture-perfect set-up where we actually had a nice house to rent rather than living somewhere weird. That's probably when we started to get more honest and transparent with each other because we knew each other's habits and pet peeves by then and were feeling braver.

'We had to talk about what we each felt OK with because Rachel was more comfortable with PDA than me and loved chatting about sex. Like, her and her boyfriend were open about using toys and would go in the shower together all the time while I was home, and I just had to remind her that it wasn't only her house. She did become more aware and, instead of lying on the sofa taking up all the room, they'd go to her room and do that there instead. But I did keep having to pull her up on stuff.

'She's the type of person to use all the hot water up on a bath that she sits in for two hours, but would be the first person to make you a cup of tea when you get home. I think, because I knew how kind she was and I benefited from that as a friend, the niggles around the house didn't bother me so much. It's like recognising each other's pitfalls but also their qualities, and realising that they balance out – or, at least, what they bring to your life is more valuable than what they do to annoy you.

'Our intention was always, "We're going to make this work", and I think it allowed us to be negative when we needed to be. I could be annoyed with her, but I loved her. You have to be able to be honest. We aren't very argumentative people, but we are very emotional people, so we would confide in each other a lot if we were upset about something or each other. Usually, one of us would cry and then the other one would be like, "Oh" and then we'd figure it out together. We celebrated lots of small wins in those years, too – there was a lot of Prosecco. We were both still finding our way in the world, and in London, and we were each other's home in a way.'

I'm struck by Hayley's honest approach and how it allowed her and Rachel to live side by side and grow, while also honouring the friendship that was at the centre of their living situation for that time. I never felt brave enough to be so open in my friendship with Phoebe in our house share.

I wish Phoebe or I had had the words to properly work through that problematic period of our time living together. Or, like Hayley and Rachel, we'd set more of a concrete intention and held our friendship at the heart of all that came our way. Or, like Hannah, we'd had the conversation when it wasn't working and called it a day before our friendship was broken beyond repair.

We live with friends because we know them, care about them, have fun with them. When it goes well, it's nurturing and fun. But we need to acknowledge that there will be bumps along the way and be ready to work through them.

I ask Dr Sandra Wheatley, a chartered social psychologist with a special interest in relationships, what does conscious cohabiting look like when you're living with friends?

'To be open and honest at every twist and turn. Your friendship will continually form and re-form throughout the time you're living together, and throughout the rest of your lives. Try to remember what encouraged your friendship to flower and do more of it – not just to maintain the friendship but to allow it to grow and develop.

'Ask yourself, as many times and as often as you need to: "Am I going to let this take the shine off our friendship?" It might take a great deal of reminding yourself that the irritation you're feeling is situational, but it'll pay off. Then, make a decision that you're both going to do your damnedest while you live together not to let house share things ruin your friendship, and to put the effort in.'

Friendship therapy

Phoebe and I lived together for another year in the Balham house share after Ben finally disappeared. In that time, I observed her slowly healing while the tension Ben had created in the house subsided and the usual rhythm of the flat started to return. A new housemate arrived and, in many ways, it felt like a new beginning. There were house dinners, evening outings, and day trips to the coast. We moved forward without addressing what had occurred: Phoebe and I wordlessly committed to a 'pretend it never happened and carry on' approach.

But the unresolved conflict in our relationship resurfaced six months later – a year and a half after Ben's departure. We were at the tail end of the Covid pandemic and, this time, it was me who made bad choices that had an impact on the house.

Lockdown was over, but Covid anxieties in the house were still running high, so we agreed collectively that we would continue to meet people outdoors rather than indoors. But one night, I had too much to drink and went into my friend's house. I had broken our pact and my housemates' trust. When I got home, it was Phoebe who pulled me up for it. I was defensive, not wanting to admit that I'd messed up. I was also outraged that she dared to do this after all we'd endured because of her relationship with Ben. I'd stuck to the 'pretend it never happened and carry on' contract that I thought we had between us, and I was incensed that she wasn't doing the same.

In one long monologue, I unleashed everything that I'd been holding on to. As is typical when you don't address small niggles at the time they arise, the dams burst and I gave her an unfiltered, honest account of what I thought – that she'd been a terrible friend, never addressing what had happened. We never resolved it and by the time I moved out to live with Noah, I was exhausted by the tension between us. We didn't speak for two years. There have been conversations since – attempts to paper over the cracks – but the trouble is that, when you live together, you see a side of someone and you can't forget it. For us, the cracks were too deep to ever be repaired.

I look back on our time living together with sadness now, unable to hold on to the happy memories without feeling a tinge of regret. I wonder whether I could have tried harder to protect our friendship in the face of events we never saw coming.

There is little awareness of how to deal with a friendship in crisis but it feels as though that's about to change. Books unpicking the foundations of friendship have been coming thick and fast: *Friendaholic* by Elizabeth Day, *BFF?* by Claire Cohen, and *Big Friendship* by Aminatou Sow and Ann Friedman. Each of them addresses the fact that we don't always have the language to rationalise or position friends in our lives. Instead, we lean on the lexicon used for family, but these words don't encompass the complexity of friendship or acknowledge that friendship is different and based on choice.

Also, in the past five years or so, friendship therapy – when two friends see a therapist together to seek mediation or coaching – has risen in popularity.[8] I ask a friendship therapist, counsellor, and director of the Baltimore Therapy Centre, Raffi Bilek, for his insights into what happened between Phoebe and me and what he might have suggested if we'd worked with him at the time to resolve our conflict.

'Friendship therapy follows a similar framework to couples counselling, in the sense that it's helping two people manage the relationship between them and get things to where they want to be,' Raffi says. 'It's a little different but, in many ways, the dynamics are the same. You care, the relationship is important to you, you want to listen, and you want to do things differently to improve the relationship.

'One thing to say about your friendship is that it is a lot easier to disconnect and take space from a friendship when you don't live together. That definitely makes a difference. In your case, it sounds like there was a very close friendship. If you'd come to me, I would have worked with you both to acknowledge that there are things to be discussed. So, we would get really clear on the fact that there was a problem between you and establish that you both wanted to work it out. And then it would be about gaining the skills to be able to do that.

'It sounds like the reason that things didn't get discussed is because you were afraid of what would happen if you were honest about how you felt. Maybe you were worried about a reaction or about losing the friendship if you asked for what you needed. So, I would help you with the skills and the tools to have a conversation about those difficult things.

'It's about being clear what we want from the relationship. All relationships have bumps in the road but, even then, you can still feel connected and like you're on the same team, as opposed to arguing, pushing, and jockeying for position. I would bring out the things that are going on for you both now as well as the underlying things you might be sitting on. We'd go back through the earlier incidents that caused you anxiety and try to unburden those things. To share them in a way that strengthens the relationship. The truth is, everybody needs help in their relationships. I don't think people realise that friendship therapy is a thing, but I think if there was more awareness, it would save so many friendships.'

And, as communications professor and close relationship researcher Emily Langan says, 'From their initiation through their evolution, relationships take work. Close relationships such as friendships and marriages can be voluntarily initiated and terminated. As such, the vitality of any relationship depends upon strategic and routine maintenance efforts. Maintenance may take different forms and functions, depending upon the goals of the partners, and research indicates that maintaining relationships is important both for the individuals and their relationship… I have studied the development and significance of friendship and its unique role from other relationships, such as kin or romantic associations.

Friendship, as a relationship type, does not appear stable throughout the life course. In other words, the relationship's value and role take on different values at different stages of life.'[9]

I hold on to the idea of 'strategic and routine maintenance efforts' that Emily outlines and to Raffi's observation that it is possible to stay connected to a friend and on the same team while navigating bumps in the road. I realise that this is what Hayley implemented when she was living with her school friend Rachel. The purpose for their friendship was clear: they were emotionally available to each other, sharing what upset them, maintaining an equilibrium, but also reassessing their priorities at every turn and leaving room for them to expand and grow as their friendship took on different roles at different times.

There are, I think, some friends who are up to the challenge of living together – but both of you need to enter into it with your eyes wide open. I also think that there are some personality types who aren't able to make it work. It's vital to be as honest as possible with each other about how compatible you are. When it works, it can – as Hayley attested – be the best thing. When it doesn't, as a pair, you can discuss if it would be best for the friendship to stop living together. Either way, the key is to be proactive, face up to the risk you're taking, and commit to making the necessary effort to keep the friendship afloat. Living with a friend cost me a friendship, but this doesn't have to be the outcome for you.

Chapter reflections
How can you ensure that you decide rather than slide into living together?
Before living with a friend, make sure you have a frank and open discussion about what you each hope to get out of it, how you will navigate prioritising the friendship, and what will happen if it doesn't work out. Make sure it feels like

a conscious decision rather than a casual arrangement in which you're just hoping for the best. Even if it's a short and temporary arrangement, it's worth scoping out your expectations for how it's going to be ahead of making a decision one way or the other.

Set an intention
Like Hayley and Rachel, can you set an intention for your time living together? It might be that you both see it as a temporary base for a year, but it might be that you're hoping to live together for a few years and give your friendship the opportunity to grow, to try new things together.

Honour the roots of your friendship
Can you find an activity to do together that involves you both bringing the version of yourself that led to the forming of the friendship in the first place? Perhaps it's something you'd always do when you didn't live together – seeing a film or attending a book club or exhibition together. Whatever it is, you're giving space to what led to you becoming friends, which will help you to separate the friendship from anything causing conflict in the house share.

What maintenance efforts can you see yourself responding well to when it comes to protecting your friendship?
You can decide on these up front, but if you're already living together, it's not too late to suggest implementing something that allows you both to make sure you're still on the same page. It might be that you're very good at tuning in to each other emotionally and you naturally share what's upsetting you. If that's the case, agree that you will both try not to take being pulled up for bad habits or household issues personally. If you're less likely to share your irritations openly along the way, can you make sure that the two of you meet for a coffee once a month to

air any frustrations that have arisen? You could even agree on some specific topics to cover ahead of time. It might feel a bit forced asking, 'So, how are you feeling in the house at the moment?' but it's worth opening up the opportunity to have that conversation so you can work on issues together and nip them in the bud.

How can you handle differentiation effectively?

Can you find a way to make room for your differences instead of hiding or denying them? If you can face these and discuss them, you can stay emotionally close while also being open and honest. To do this well, you need to accept a level of constructive criticism from your housemates so you get familiar with your strengths and weaknesses. Can you think what these might be, based on previous house shares or feedback from friends?

How can you separate housemate issues from friendship issues?

You've probably heard this said to romantic couples: 'Don't let a housemate issue become a relationship issue.' It's an important distinction to make when you're living with a friend too. It enables you to categorise things like bad washing-up habits or not emptying the washing machine under 'housemate problems' and not let them threaten your friendship, which is, in reality, more valuable to you than a pristine home. It also means that you might feel more comfortable addressing those small housemate issues as what they are, simply asking people to tidy up after themselves, rather than thinking of them as personal attacks on your friend.

4. Rupture and repair

How to handle housemate conflict

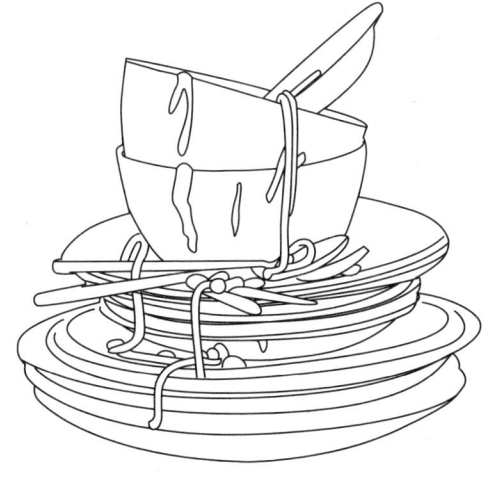

"Every relationship is at risk of moments of frustration or as the term has it, of 'rupture'... Repair refers to the work needed for two people to regain each other's trust"

Alain de Botton[1]

I have only once let my emotions and frustrations build up to a state that we house sharers should try to avoid at all costs: boiling point.

I'm standing in the lounge of my Balham house share, where Phoebe and I have lived together for three years. I'm delivering The Monologue to Phoebe and I can feel myself shaking. No detail's gone unshared, not to do with her boyfriend Ben's bad behaviour, him betraying our trust, or how she'd let it go on for too long. I don't pause once to think or even breathe as I itemise the things that I believe she should have done better to protect our friendship. I'm being ruthless and I can feel myself going too far, but I can't stop.

I finish speaking. I can't believe what I've just said. Words revealing my most private thoughts have detonated in the air between us. Phoebe's saying nothing; she's just looking at me, visibly hurt. The veneer that we were putting on our friendship has shattered to reveal the mess beneath.

I'm crying. I take a deep breath and walk to my room. I gently press the door shut, sit on my bed, and think, 'Fuck.' I feel sick, regretting the way things came out. Phoebe knocks on my door. She's crying too.

'I'm sorry. I really don't want us to fall out,' I say.

'Me neither, Al,' she says. We sit on the edge of my bed and hug and things feel a little better.

In the days that follow, our normal daily routines resume, slightly altered by the tension between us. We smile when we pass each other on the landing and, when we're both in the kitchen cooking, we make small talk about our days and weekend plans. But there's a flatness to our exchanges. As I wait for our friendship to return to what it was, the tension is like a weight and it's getting heavier. I think about it when I wake up, dreading bumping into her in the kitchen over breakfast. I think about it the whole commute home from work, worried about what the vibe will be in the house that evening. Because our 10-year-friendship is on the line, I can't stop it playing on my mind.

I think of another time when I faced conflict in a house share – this time with a housemate called Annie, who I lived with in an earlier house share in Balham and met through SpareRoom. In the first two months we lived together, she had been quite short with me, telling me and the other two housemates that we weren't making her feel welcome. When she asked about subletting her room so she could go travelling for a month and we said we'd rather she didn't, she was so angry, she sent a stream of aggressive texts and stopped speaking to us. In the aftermath, there was discomfort and an awkwardness whenever we were in the same room, but this didn't play on my mind in quite the same way as the scenario with Phoebe did. Conflict in house shares comes in many forms and, whoever you're living with, a sense of unease in your living space is all-encompassing. Especially when you're not equipped with tools to remedy it.

I look back on these situations now, as a seasoned house sharer, and try to see the actual conflict as a small portion of the issue at hand. A rupture is bound to occur at some point – a natural by-product of when adults with opinions and preferences live together – so it's something I should try not to attach too much meaning to or dwell on. If the actual conflict is 10 per cent of the issue, the other 90 per cent is the repair. It's the repair we should focus on because that's the bit we can control and learn to do better.

Rupture and repair

A concept rooted in attachment theory, British psychiatrist and psychoanalyst John Bowlby developed the theory of rupture and repair in 1958. Seeing how he breaks down the cycle of disconnection (rupture) and restoration (repair) in close relationships[2] helps me to untangle past housemate conflicts that I've experienced.

Bowlby shows the various ways that conflicts arise in relationships and how they unfold. Each pathway begins the same – with a conflict – but unfolds differently and has different outcomes. His theory outlines three possible directions in which a conflict can go. On the first pathway, a conflict occurs and there's an initial disconnection (an argument). That's followed by a state of tension (when you're a bit shitty with each other post the argument) and then, in the third stage along this pathway, the disconnection is repaired (you make up), the tension lifts, and the relationship is restored. You move forwards, stronger.

For the second pathway, after the initial disconnection occurs (an argument), you remain disconnected, or 'ruptured' and, as a result, you live with a tension that doesn't shift and you continue being shitty with each other.

On the third pathway, the initial disconnection (the argument) causes the relationship to end.

So, looking at this cycle and the pathways, there are three possible outcomes when a disconnection or disconnection and rupture occur: we navigate the tension and effect a repair, so a rupture is avoided; no repair is found, so we remain in a state of tension; or the relationship ends.

Repairing a relationship after a conflict (whether there's been a rupture or not), requires tools. Without them, housemates either have to live with the tension or their relationship collapses. It's why so many people leave a house share when they hit a rough patch with one or more of their housemates. It's what I did after a long period living alongside Phoebe in a fog of tension that didn't shift.

Passionate about the sustainability potential of co-living, Dr Penny Clark co-founded a consultancy to help shared living communities and businesses thrive. She researches shared living spaces and has visited a range of co-living spaces and intentional communities. I ask her what she's observed about conflict in co-living spaces and how this might apply to a house share. 'You've got to be able to be real with people in a way that's still compassionate and respectful', she says. 'Because if you constantly deny what you need and push it down, then, in the end, you'll just want to move out or you might end up getting really angry. Or your housemate might do something tiny and then that's the thing you react to. It's about understanding your own feelings and needs, which will enable you to be real with someone about what it is and what you need, even if it feels insignificant.'

I've seen people reach boiling point in house shares, too, and it is usually because they have done exactly this – pushed down annoyances for too long and then they've erupted. This was, I think, why Annie felt the need to send aggressive texts and stop talking to me and the other housemates when we said we didn't want her to sublet her room.

In another house share I lived in, there was a heated discussion with a different housemate – this time because she thought my housemate and I were slamming doors deliberately loudly to piss her off. In the end, she decided to leave the house share without saying anything, reporting us to the landlord for having a pet rabbit, and emptying the contents of our cutlery drawer, which she either took with her or disposed of somewhere. We never discovered which, but she didn't even leave us a teaspoon to stir our cups of tea.

Those who do manage to stay cool about such things often do so by releasing some passive-aggressive energy along the way. We've all been on the receiving end of those Post-it notes and WhatsApps. Learning how to field them is as much a rite of passage as getting the key to your first house share.

Between the bills, cleanliness, noise, and visiting policies, house shares are a breeding ground for conflicts of all kinds. In house shares, I've witnessed every single one that psychologists have identified: differences in opinion over how a task should be done (task conflict), differences in personality (relationship conflict), and differences in values, politics, and religion (value conflict).[3] I've lost count of the number of times I've heard the phrase, 'We fell out when we were living together.' This happens because, without the tools and self-awareness we need to handle living alongside others in a house share, many of us reach the point of no return.

Priya Isaacs, 31, a doctor from Islington, can't see a way out of the conflict in her house share other than to leave. She wasn't ever very close to her housemates, but they got along fine before there was a disagreement about the bills. Now, things are really difficult. 'It's hard,' she says. 'It's really weird and really unnatural to live in a house with someone and not talk to them. Since having a disagreement with my housemates over the bills, I've just made a lot of plans to be out the house to compensate. I have tried to talk to one of my housemates, but he doesn't understand how it's really upset me, and we just end up disagreeing again. So there's a really uncomfortable atmosphere in the house. Is there anything to be gained from me communicating how I feel? At this point, I'm genuinely thinking I'm just going to move out.'

When things have become fraught with resentment and conflict in a house share, it maybe does feel like there is no reason to attempt some sort of reconciliation. If the person you're clashing with doesn't seem like your type of person anyway and you can't see yourself staying in touch with them, it's understandable that you might not want to make an effort to build a better relationship with them. I've certainly reached that point in several house shares. But that led me to move eight times, spending a lot of money on renting vans, and feeling perpetually unsettled.

There is some middle ground, though, on which house sharers – me included – should be brave enough to tread, which is to aim at establishing a functional, *good enough* relationship. This person doesn't ever have to be your best friend, so you've got nothing to lose. Take the risk, have the difficult conversation with them about how you can make the relationship better for the time you're living together. If you like the house, your room, and the location, it is at least worth trying to build a relationship that works, even if it isn't one you see going the distance. Moving out is always still an option, but there is another: repair the relationship.

Finding a framework

Conflict at home is not something that's specific to a house share. It happens all the time in families and couples living together. But what a house share lacks – which families or couples are more likely to have access to – is a framework for understanding and navigating disagreements.

I lived with a partner for two and a half years and, during that time, as most couples do at some stage, we experienced all the types of conflict noted earlier in this chapter – namely, task, relationship, and value. But because we had mapped out a road ahead that, at the time, we were both committed to staying on, we were hugely invested in understanding these conflicts, looking at them closely, interrogating them, and finding better ways to deal with them. At one point, we even took ourselves to couples therapy, where we sat on a couch and a nice lady handed us a printed piece of paper and on it were the stages that all couples go through, including times of conflict and crisis.[4] I remember feeling hugely validated and relieved that it wasn't just us struggling with this stuff – it was every couple. There it was, neatly laid out in a shiny leaflet: a framework, like a flowchart, that explained what stage we were in and what conflicts might arise, plus tools for resolving them. Though, in the end, our differences were too great to work through and the relationship ended, I found the framework itself so helpful, then and since.

I learned that there are six stages in a romantic relationship. First, there's symbiosis or bonding, when two people, with different interests and lives, come together and form an attachment to one another. Usually at this point, the couple is focusing on the similarities as their two separate lives merge. Next, there's the differentiation phase, which the couples therapist I saw told me is when most couples come to see her – struggling to handle the differences they've discovered between them.

Within the differentiation phase, there's a spectrum. Those who are less well equipped to deal with eachothers' differences might find themselves either assuming that their partner knows how they feel without them actually saying anything or expressing how they feel with frustration. Those who are better at allowing for eachothers' differences are able to see things from their partner's point of view, to share their thoughts and feelings, and to trust that their partner will receive what they say well. These partners are often able to navigate their differences in a healthy way and any tensions they might bring to a relationship.

Allowing for others' differences is difficult and even more so when you live together in close quarters – so we were handed even more leaflets that explained the differentiation stage in more detail and how to practise doing it well as a couple. These included ideas for role play, with scripts for each of us, and tips on how to take a timeout and improve how you argue. All these tools were ready and waiting for couples to learn about and implement to better how they manage tensions in their relationships.

There's a reason why a framework exists for cohabiting partners: because living alongside each other while maintaining a healthy relationship takes work. But more of us are house sharing and for longer periods of time than ever before,[5] so we need a similar framework for housemates. Not having one only exacerbates any conflicts that arise. And when they happen, we are staring at a blank page, not sure where to go next. If there were such a thing for house sharers, it would help us to see how, as housemates, we can deal with and move through conflicts, so we could learn how to repair our relationships with them, which might stop us from feeling like the only option is to move out. I hope that, in the future, there are therapists specialising in house share conflict resolution.

In today's world, though, it doesn't help that, socially, housemate relationships aren't given enough recognition. When I've had conflicts with friends or arguments with a boyfriend, friends and family have weighed in readily with their own experiences, and we've spent hours thinking them over and working out what could be done better. However, whenever I've needed to talk about my housemate relationships, conversations aren't as rich. I've noticed that others don't have the same capacity to care, tolerance to listen, or willingness to give advice. Because, historically, house sharing has been a very temporary situation, we haven't been taught just how important these relationships are. As a result, there is no framework for how to resolve conflict in them.

Yet, for the time we are living with them, the relationships with our housemates are just as significant as those in any other home set-up you might find – and potentially just as detrimental to our mental wellbeing. As you and I know, housemates are important. They have a huge impact on our lives. We can learn a lot along the way if we take the time to nurture our relationships with them.

And the lessons learned from understanding where conflict comes from and how to resolve it will never be wasted.

Once we change our mindset and acknowledge that the housemate relationship is one that does have an impact on our day-to-day life and wellbeing, we can find the motivation and time to work at it, even if we're not wanting to be friends but just to live alongside one another in peace. When you are housemates, there is a connection that needs an appropriate level of attention. And a framework.

How to resolve conflict in your house share: a seven-step framework

Step 1: Observe

When some tension or frustration occurs, take a step back to look at and process it. Write it down or talk it out with someone close to you. Work out how much of the frustration is down to your mood or personal preference. In her book *It's On Me*, existential psychotherapist Dr Sara Kuburic – Instagram's Millennial Therapist – explores how we can take more responsibility for our feelings. I ask her how this could be beneficial in a house share situation.

'To be able to have a healthy and helpful conversation with a housemate, you need to know the role you played in the disagreement. One of my favourite pieces of advice is "find your 5 per cent". Maybe your housemate is 95 per cent in the wrong. But find and acknowledge the 5 per cent or even find and accept the half a per cent that you contributed. You probably contributed in some way.'

Accepting our responsibility like this can stop resentment from building. As Sara says, 'If you put all the blame on your housemate, you're going to hold negative thoughts and feelings that will fuel resentment. That resentment will likely bleed into every conversation you have with your housemate – you're going to get into an endless cycle of talking to your friends about it, and you're going to make your housemate the villain and you're going to become the victim.'

Taking time to observe, notice, and interrogate a frustration before initiating a conversation gives you a chance to look at the part you played.

Step 2: Initiate

If you're the one highlighting something with your housemate, be vulnerable. Begin with your feelings and share how it is affecting you. And, before you start the conversation, be really clear on exactly what it is you want to say.

'Before talking or bringing an issue up, figure out what you're upset about,' says Sara. 'The problem is that lots of people process and gain awareness *while* they speak, so they will immediately go up to their housemate (without processing first) and try to pinpoint what's going on for them during the conversation. This can confuse the housemate and introduce conflict.'

Sara gives the example of someone getting frustrated at their housemate for leaving food out in the kitchen. But, actually, they're not only annoyed about the food being left out, they're also annoyed about the fact that their space isn't being respected, previous requests have been ignored, and they feel like they are carrying the mental load of the house. 'It's important to know what you're angry about before communicating it. People don't do this enough,' she says.

Step 3: Enquire

If your housemate is pulling you up on something, now's the time to be curious and ask questions. Your aim in this scenario is to understand more about your housemate and the issue they're raising. Look at the bigger picture and, remember, it's not personal.

Sara recommends reflective listening: 'As your housemate is talking to you, instead of talking back right away, make sure you actually know what they're saying (rather than just thinking about what you want to say next). Say something like, "What I am hearing you say is…" or "What I sense from what you've said is…" Then, in your own words, reflect what they just said. For example, "My understanding of why you're upset about is… is this correct?" It makes the other person feel heard and avoids misunderstandings. A lot of conflict escalates because people feel unseen, unheard, not valued, not justly treated. The second you go, "Here's your spotlight. I'm listening. I care enough to try and understand you", a lot of conflict de-escalates.'

Step 4: Focus

Focus on the difference between you that's causing the friction, and don't make it personal. 'If you start telling your housemate that they're lazy, unreliable, sloppy or messy, you're just triggering conflict,' says Sara. 'Give your housemate a specific problem and target it (dirty dishes or overnight guests, for example).' Phrase it in a way that lets them know you want to work together to create a better home environment. So, you might say, 'X is getting me down, can we change such and such habit or behaviour?'

Step 5: Regulate

Stay in tune with your own emotions and stress levels as much as you can. If you feel yourself getting closer to boiling point, breathe, get a glass of water, or ask to have a timeout. This might be a useful window of opportunity for you if you're conflict averse or need a bit of time to process things. Some people are quick on their feet in conversations and others need time to think before they respond.

If you need to take a break from a difficult discussion, just make sure that you offer an explanation and promise of a return to it. Take a timeout responsibly and intentionally. Avoid leaving the conversation without communicating what you're doing. Try,

'This conversation doesn't seem to be getting us anywhere, let's take a break.' Make a commitment to resume the discussion, too, such as, 'Shall we go for a coffee in the morning and talk about it more then?'

'People take timeouts all the time in house shares, but they'll go to their own rooms and just avoid common areas without explaining why,' says Sara. 'Saying something snarky and going into your room and slamming your door isn't a timeout, it's a tantrum. And that can be really toxic. If you feel like you're going in circles or that you're having a hard time processing or coming up with a solution, suggest a pause and then a time to pick the conversation back up. A timeout is a deliberate space you take by announcing its purpose and telling them when you're going to resume.'

Step 6: Reflect

During a timeout or after a difficult conversation, try to structure your thoughts, feelings, and reflections in a constructive way. It can stop unhelpful rumination, which can sometimes worsen your feelings towards a conflict. To help you to think constructively about the different aspects of conflict, reflect on these questions.

• What just happened and what did it feel like? What was your immediate emotional response? How did you behave? What else were you feeling? Is there anything in your history that might have been triggered?
• What was happening for your housemate? What in their history might have come to the surface?
• How would you have liked it to have gone? Do you wish they'd stayed calmer? Do you wish they'd listened more intently?
• What's happening right now? Could an acknowledgement, a hug, a conversation, or an apology help to resolve the incident? What do you need? What might your housemate need?

Step 7: Repair

Being clear in your mind about what happened, what you wish had gone differently, and your desired outcome is a good foundation for repair. Ask what the other person needs from you to get back on track. Hopefully, they will ask the same; if not, offer it yourself. Sara suggests some repair phrases:

- 'I've been reflecting on X and I realise that was totally on me. I just want to apologise. It won't happen again.'
- 'I know I've messed up pretty badly. I understand that your trust might be broken. I want to apologise. I am sorry. My behaviour was inappropriate, and I should have spoken with you about X, Y, or Z. What can I do to repair our relationship?'
- 'What do you need to see from me so we can start to rebuild the trust between us?'
- Followed by, 'This is what I think I need…' Then, give it time.

Beyond the surface

One of the biggest stumbling blocks is that, as humans, we don't always give one another enough background knowledge. If we did offer a wider context or our workings out, it might help others to understand our behaviour. If, as housemates, we can achieve the necessary fine balance, sharing an appropriate amount about what's happening for us internally, I think it would help us to make sense of the conflicts that arise. But to do this takes self-reflection, empathy, and good communication skills.

When we face conflict in a house share, it usually comes down to four questions.

- What are you bringing?
- What are they bringing?
- How can you have a conversation that makes room for what you're both bringing?
- How can you work together to resolve the issue at hand?

I tested this out recently on the seed of a difficulty that was taking root in my new house share. I'd only been living there for two weeks, which happened to be the coldest weeks of the year. During that time, I was working at home, so wanted to put the heating on, but my housemate was going out to work every day. I asked a couple of times if it was OK for me to put the heating on, but sensed there was a little bit of apprehension. I was getting stressed about it because, having had my own place before, I was used to being in control of these decisions. In my own flat, I'd been in charge of the bills, knew how much things cost, and could weigh up the cost-to-comfort ratio. Here, it's my housemate who's in charge of all that.

But it turned out that these worries were based on my own stuff, not the actual situation. In the end, I explained to my housemate that I was worried about putting the heating on. It gave her an opportunity to share that the previous housemate had cranked the heating up all day while she was at work and it caused a rift between them. I explained that I understood it would be unfair for her to have to pay more because of me and said I was happy to increase my contribution towards the bills if necessary. We resolved it, making room for her stuff and my stuff. She needed reassurance that I wasn't going to do what the other housemate did and I needed the heating on.

More often than not, as in this case, there is something occurring beneath the surface, and I think we need to be able to share that when we are cohabiting. It is what shapes our behaviour and helps us as humans to be more understanding of one another.

Social scientist Dr Penny Clark reiterates this point, having visited a number of communities and co-living spaces in the course of her research. 'Self-awareness is really important,' she says. 'It's tricky living with people. People do things that really annoy us. And sometimes people annoy us. And we think that it's because of X but, actually, it's Y. And maybe Y is actually not really to do with them; maybe it's because you had a really bad day or what they did happened to trigger a past bad incident in your mind. Being able to really understand and reflect on what you need and how you feel is a really useful skill for living with others.

'Something I learned during researching co-living and an approach I'm really keen on is non-violent communication. It has helped me a lot. It was developed in the 1960s by a psychologist called Marshall Rosenberg and it has been used in everything from anti-racism to diplomacy to helping husbands and wives understand each other better. Instead of seeing people or situations as right and wrong, you try to look at humans as having certain needs and wanting to fulfil those needs. It means understanding your own needs at the same time as understanding the needs of others. It provides some frameworks for making requests of people that otherwise would be quite difficult conversations to have, so it can really help with conflict. But it's not just about that – it offers a different way of seeing the world.

'So just one example of non-violent communication being really effective is two housemates I visited where one was having a problem because the other was closing doors loudly after 10pm. When the person who was closing the doors first heard this, they were a bit reactive: "Oh, for goodness sake, it's a bit much. I just want to be able to close the doors. Why is this a big deal?" But then the person who was finding the doors being closed too loudly explained that they find it very hard to sleep – they've always been a light sleeper. Things were happening in their life, which meant that it was difficult for them to feel well rested. And when these doors were closing loudly, it was waking them up. And in non-violent communication, you're meant to explain "This is the need I have." So the need actually is not to close the door quietly; the need is, "I need rest, I need good rest." And then you explain the request, which is, "Please, can you close the doors quietly?" And the person who heard this no longer felt reactive. They were happy to be more mindful about the doors because they understood that this person just wanted good rest. Whereas, before, they didn't understand why the other person might feel a bit annoyed by it, by explaining the situation, they avoided degrading their relationship.'

It comes down to communicating an appropriate amount of what's happening beneath the surface to those you're living with. Being able to think about the need that's behind your request helps everyone to reach an understanding and avoid feeling completely overwhelmed and annoyed. It's only natural that you won't want to overshare, especially if your housemate is someone you've just met. You want to create a healthy amount of distance, not hear all the inner workings of your housemate's mind. But imagine if, on entering a house share, we could have a frank conversation and talk through our 'housemate CV', detailing what housemates need to know about one another. A bit like a more in-depth dating profile, it would include a neat summary of our vulnerabilities, pet peeves, fears, triggers, how we deal with conflict, what helps us to repair after a conflict, and what makes us feel calm. But without this, it's down to us to share enough about ourselves to provide the necessary context for those we're living with.

Creating a time and forum to air thoughts, feelings, and frustrations can be really powerful. It's something my ex-partner and I did on the advice of our couples therapist, and something I know other couples living together do too. Choose an evening a week to chat about how you're feeling in the house. It's an opportunity to raise things you're worried about or that have bothered you. If, as a house share, you can agree to check in with one another on a weekly or a monthly basis to air frustrations, this might help you all to deal with things as they arise, so they don't fester or have a chance to come to a head.

In her research, Penny has observed that such regular meetings in communities give everyone a chance to voice frustrations. 'For the vast majority of people, the idea of having a weekly meeting or monthly meeting feels sort of like work. And people don't want to put rules on each other either or formalise agreements because that just doesn't feel comfortable. If you're quite extrovert, and comfortable expressing yourself, you probably don't need those structures to communicate the things you need to share. However, if maybe you find it hard to raise things or you might describe yourself as more introverted, having a bit of structure in place, like having a moment when you can raise something that you think is important, can be helpful. Without that structure there, you might not feel you can raise it.'

Me, myself, and conflict

An integral part of being able to communicate clearly and concisely what's going on underneath the surface for you is knowing what this is yourself. If you get to a point where you feel comfortable and clear on your needs and what happens for you when you experience conflict, you will better understand your discomfort when it arises, be better at reading others' reactions, and use this knowledge to inform constructive conversations with your housemates.

'Everyone struggles with conflict. Yet, we're not taught how to sidestep unnecessary conflict or what to do when we're in it,' says Sara. 'However, millennial women seem to have very strong people-pleasing tendencies – the "good girl tendency", the "just buckle up and do it" tendency that was taught and is expected. I'm noticing that millennial women don't have that impulse (or permission) or that confidence to stand up for themselves. And so often, when faced with conflict, they're trying to make sure the other person walks away feeling happy and not mad at them. They act from a place of "How do I make sure this person doesn't hate me?" rather than "Is this problem actually resolved? Did I get what I need?" Those are questions I generally don't hear millennial women asking themselves.'

Sara's observations certainly map on to what I have found in my conversations with women who are house sharing. They have said that they struggle to ask for what they need as they are too concerned about being disliked.

In her book *It's On Me,* Sara explores how we can take more responsibility for getting what we need to feel fulfilled. Part of this is understanding why we behave like we do when conflict arises. Sara talks about how each of us has an innate tendency to respond in a certain way to conflict, subconsciously adopting one of four coping reactions, or reflexes, to protect ourselves: distancing, overactivity, aggression, or freezing.

'These are reflexive boundaries,' she says when I ask her about them, meaning that they're automatic responses. 'You set them subconsciously, so you won't always notice how your need is violated because it's not like someone crossing a conscious boundary we have set. You will just notice that you feel uneasy, hurt, or resentful. It's an automatic coping reaction that helps you feel safe. It's different for each of us. If distancing is your tendency, you might walk out of the house. If aggression is your tendency, you might make a sarcastic joke. If it's freezing, you might find yourself feeling stunned and not able to reply. If overactivity is your tendency, you might find ways to stay busy to avoid the conversation or (on the opposite end of the spectrum) want to talk about things all the time. Whatever your tendency is, you'll feel an urge to do it. And you might see it in your housemates, too. Understanding your tendency is key, not just because it will help you to understand when you're triggered, but because it will help you get your needs met in a way that's more conducive to living harmoniously with other people.'

When I look at the conflicts I've experienced in house shares, I can see that my reflex is aggression. But that doesn't always look like reaching boiling point. Sometimes it has manifested as feeling like a situation was so unjust that I needed to call my sister and rant at her down the phone, or tidy something up, hoping the person would get the message that I was annoyed they'd left their things out. As Sara outlines in her book, 'Unlike sadness, which often wants to hide, anger evokes a sense of self-expression. Aggression typically emerges from a deep sense of powerlessness and leads to a desire to "run down" (destroy) the threat. When the aggressive impulse is combined with a sense of "justice", meaning we feel we have the "right" to lash out, we begin to punish others. It's a way to harm the offender in order to offset the injustice (vengeance). It's also about "teaching" someone a lesson, even if that someone is us. Aggression is not always obvious.'[6]

Knowing my own boundary reflex, I started to be more aware of when things crossed and triggered it. Usually, what made me feel vulnerable was something small that left me powerless – like not being able to put the heating on while working at home. By learning how to use the tools I needed to express that feeling before my aggresssion reflex kicked in, I was able to work with that reflex rather than ignore it.

Those times when my behaviour during a conflict caused a rupture, I was left feeling embarrassed that I'd let something get to me. I felt that I'd behaved unkindly and didn't really know what to do to make it better.

'When it comes to repair, my go to is words and actions,' says Sara. 'Try saying something like, "I've been reflecting on such and such and I realise that was totally on me. I just want to apologise." You can also just not do it again. An apology without changed behaviour is not an apology. Sometimes we screw up so badly. Maybe you went in their room without asking or promised a room to someone else. Then all you can do is say, "Hey, I screwed up pretty badly. I understand that maybe your trust might be broken. I want to apologise, I'm so sorry. That was inappropriate and I should have consulted you. What can I do to repair this relationship? What do you need to see from me in order for us to start to rebuild the trust and the safety in our relationship?" Most people will respond well to that, and if they don't offer any tangible ways to help you repair it, then you apologise and make sure your behaviour aligns with that apology moving forward, and give it some time.'

In an ideal world, we would all be self-aware and come into a house share with solid ideas of our flaws, boundaries, and reflexes and how best to communicate them. But when there is a range of personalities, preferences, and situations in a house share, that's never going to happen. Sometimes the more aware among us have to do a little heavy lifting to keep the peace.

I ask Sara if it's helpful to understand others' reflexes, to bring context to a conflict or situation. 'It's really helpful to understand how people react and what their reflexive boundaries are,' she says. 'It's not your job to do that, but when we live with people, it might be helpful to clue in and notice they are setting up a reflexive boundary, which means something just got violated or threatened. You could even ask them. "I noticed that when I said such and such, you did this. Did that offend you? Did that hurt you or frustrate you? Can we talk about it?" It's a little bit of detective work, which I don't love to encourage people to do, because people should self-regulate and communicate. But let's be realistic, your housemate might not be self-aware and may not self-regulate. So it could be helpful to notice patterns of how they behave when they're triggered or not triggered, and then try to not violate their boundary, or ask them what's going on to help you understand the situation. The hard truth is that poor communication is not a personality trait. Poor communication comes down to lack of skill. So, yes, we can be uncomfortable having difficult conversations, but it's just a skill we don't have yet and can gain.'

Chapter reflections
What do you find most challenging about the communal areas in a house share?
Compile a list of those things that have really been getting under your skin – even if they seem small and petty. They are contributing to a level of dissatisfaction that you have the power to overcome. After you've made your list, take each niggle and think about how,

in an ideal world, you would resolve this conflict. Even if you don't feel ready to act on it now, having that plan and knowing how you could use it to resolve your problems will help you to feel more in control. If the moment presents itself and you feel able to tackle your frustrations, then you'll already have a loose plan in place.

As a house, could you discuss how you'd like to deal with conflicts?
Discussing it as something that will inevitably arise before it does is the first step towards finding a way to better deal with such events together. Can you try a weekly or monthly meet?

Being totally honest with yourself, what would you put on your housemate profile?
Here's what I'd include on mine.

• **Your house share history** I've lived in eight different house shares and enjoy connecting with the people I live with. I want a house share where I live with people who care about me, and I care about them, but that doesn't necessarily mean living in one another's pockets. It does take me some time to settle in and warm up to the people I'm living with. I struggle sometimes to say what I need, so will often hold on to resentments and let them build up.
• **Vulnerabilities** These include feeling not in control of my environment.
• **Most irritated by...** Noise.
• **Things that help me to repair after conflict** A conversation acknowledging the conflict, followed by doing something together out of the house, like a walk or drink later that week.
• **Things that help me to feel calm** Cooking, walks, watching films together, people being honest and kind.
• **Things that help me to feel safe** Having my needs considered (I am usually fine with people coming over, but it feels good when

people check it's OK first), space to cook, and feelings of connection that also allow me room to do my own thing.

How could you communicate what's on this profile to your housemates?

In conversations with your housemates, it's probably most appropriate to give a condensed version of who you are and the vulnerabilities you bring to the table. This might sound like, 'I know that, when I'm tired, I really struggle to socialise in the house and need some peace and quiet, so then I can be a bit snappy and just need some space.' Having created your co-living card in your mind will help you to provide your housemates with some context for who you are without this feeling like an intense conversation. Communicating your points ahead of time, in a relaxed and friendly manner will mean that when you're raising a conflict or having a difficult conversation, it's likely to feel easier to talk about it because you've already done the groundwork.

Can you think of a conflict you've experienced recently?

Replay the experience in your mind and answer these questions.

- What were you bringing?
- What were they bringing?
- How could you have had a conversation that made room for both your issues?
- How might you have worked together to find a resolution that resolved the conflict?

What's in your repair kit?

Either on your own or with your housemates, think about what you need when a conflict arises – what helps you to move forward and forgive? It might be as simple as a walk and a chat about the conflict. One woman I interviewed remembers a time when a housemate brought her a can of coke from the shop as an olive branch. Maybe for you it's a hug. Maybe you need a bit of space. Make a little list. But, remember, you can always ask, 'What can I do to help rebuild our relationship?'

Can you think of a house share frustration to reflect on?
Using the questions for Step 6 under the heading 'A seven-step conflict-resolution framework for house shares' earlier in this chapter, reflect on the situation that has come to mind.

Can you write a couple of repair phrases?
Using Sara's examples to get you thinking, write down a couple of your own.

5. The pecking order

Housemate hierarchy and how to find harmony

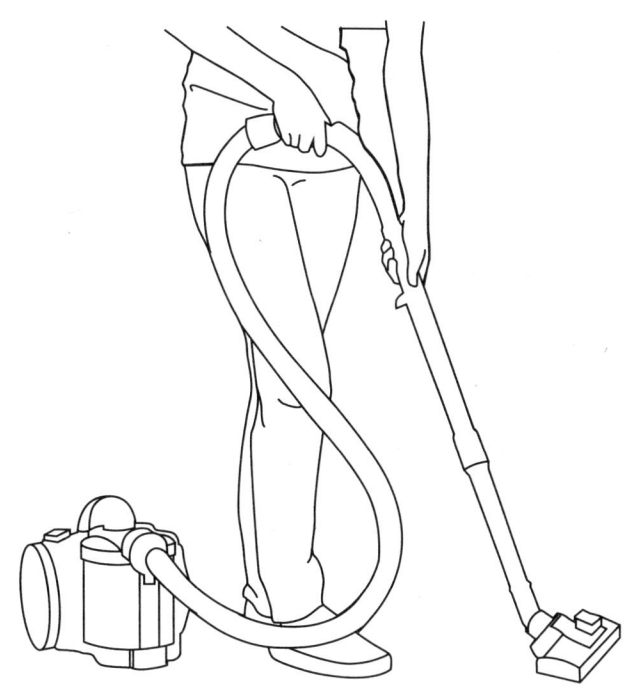

"Outer order contributes to inner calm"
Gretchen Rubin[1]

If you're house sharing, then you'll know that the real mundanities of life – household chores and cleaning – carry extra weight where communal spaces are concerned. In a shared home, these dull but necessary aspects of domestic life don't run on silently in the background. Instead, they are front and centre of housemate interactions, disagreements, and the roles played in the household. I lose track of the number of heated conversations I've had with housemates who are wound up by the politics of the shoe rack or confused by the sponge system (not everyone uses different sponges to clean the bathroom and the kitchen, it seems).

Living spaces in house shares are filled with tell-tale signs of how well bonded the housemates are or how well developed their relationships are and whether the individuals living there feel connected to the place. Having lived in eight house shares myself and visiting the people I interviewed for this book in their shared homes, I can spot the clues. A lack of cohesion in the group shows up in the cupboards full of miscellaneous items left by multiple previous housemates that have never been cleared out or broken furniture no one's thought to get rid of. But when housemates have gelled better, there are communal fruit bowls, rotas on the fridge, and homely touches, like wall art, framed photographs, a bread bin, and house plants that are fed and watered.

Compared with living in a family home or being part of a workforce where we tend to fall in with certain structures, house shares are structureless. Neither running as cohesively as a family home, nor being very functional, like a workplace, a house share sits somewhere between the two. Most of us grow up in families where there's a hierarchy with parents or carers in charge and, over time, responsibilities are allocated. There's a structure there. At school, teachers organise us into classes and groups. At work, job descriptions and those in more senior positions set out the parameters of your role, and this clear direction helps you to know what's expected and stay motivated and fulfilled.

Research shows that role ambiguity at work is linked to emotional exhaustion[2] and, for me, role ambiguity in a house share – when you don't know who makes the decisions or whether you're empowered to do certain things around the house – also results in a particular type of emotional fatigue. Without a universal structure to fall back on, we don't always naturally find our place. Continually trying to work out what's expected of you and create a sense of order in your home is exhausting.

When we do find our place and role in a house share, it's often undefined and unspoken. There's no democratic vote on who would be best at what. Instead it's more of a 'do-ocracy', with individuals, in the absence of a formal hierarchy, taking it on themselves to do a certain thing or make a decision about something that matters to them. When housemates naturally gravitate towards different tasks, a loose structure is formed in the group and, in time, those roles tend to become more defined. I've seen it happen in multiple house shares and you probably have too. You can usually spot the nurturing one, who was living in the house share first, knows the history, and shows everyone the ropes; then there's the diligent one, who's in charge of the bills;

the one who takes on the social role, getting everyone together; the one who acts as the peacemaker; and the truth teller, who never thinks twice about disrupting the status quo. Each one a valuable piece of the puzzle.

'For most of us, home is where we lived with our family and families are hierarchical,' says Jane Sassienie, a transpersonal psychotherapist whose training focuses on the interplay between the people in a group. 'So there is a kind of hardwired thing in us to recreate those hierarchies. Thinking about a house share as a space where we are recreating familial hierarchies, it makes sense that the person who got there first is the natural parent of the family.' The house share pecking order tends to be a flatter structure, though, with responsibilities and roles divvied out among those in the group. Often, the responsibilities we naturally lean in to depend on our own psychological hardwiring – the roles we played growing up and our attachment styles. Reflecting on your upbringing can help you to see how it might have shaped your expectations of what a home is for you, of those you live with, and of the role you hope to play in it.

Your personal starting point

In her book, *Every Family Has a Story,* Julia Samuel explores how our families have a profound effect on our lives and relationships. She writes, 'At the centre of our wellbeing is relationship. The quality of our lives depends on the quality of our relationships... I see that all our "relational stuff" began with our family. It is the centre of how we learn to relate to each other and how we manage emotions in every aspect of our lives – ourselves, love, friendship, work – as well as family.'[3]

I can see how my family shaped my own path, and perhaps you'll be able to see your family's influence in your house sharing journey too. Maybe you're the eldest and, as a result, you naturally take a leadership role or you had a certain role growing up that means you tend to be drawn to recreating that in your home set-up.

I grew up in a single-parent family, the youngest of three sisters. I was used to having a say in what was going on. My mum, sisters, and I would discuss what we did at the weekends, what colours we painted the walls, and what we had for dinner. With two older sisters, it was often more natural for me to assume a subordinate role, following direction and taking the path of least resistance. It meant that my focus would sometimes shift to other things, like thinking of fun things to do together, so a social role.

Sometimes I would fight to have my opinion heard. My sisters and I argued a lot, but we were also good at making up and moving on, never scared of sharing our feelings. Friends of mine still laugh now about the times they'd come over and we'd be having a screaming match – about borrowed clothes, using all the hot water, or someone playing music too loud. I always felt free to express myself. This influenced my expectations of and how I function in house shares, just as your experiences probably influence the role you take in your house shares.

'A house share coming into therapy would be so interesting,' says psychotherapist, podcaster, and author Emma Reed Turrell. 'I really believe that the roles we set up for each other and ourselves in house shares will come down to attachment theory. Our earliest attachments reincarnated in a house share.'

You may already have a loose understanding of what your own attachment style is. Formed in your early years, it's shaped by your upbringing and how your needs were met when you were young. There are four styles: anxious, avoidant, disorganised, and secure. Whichever one is yours, it can play a role in how you relate to people in your adult life. Knowing what your attachment style is and how it might play out in a house share can really help with understanding your place and relationships with others in a house share.

'Whenever we enter a new group, there's a group dynamic and

it tells us we're going to create a new "imago": a mental image of another person and our relation to them. And that is the point at which we start to place people from our past and project them on to the people in that group. So let's say you go into a new house share, you will find someone there who in the initial experience will remind you of your mum, your childhood friend, your sister. That's really normal. That's part of how groups form. Typically, we update those projections, and we start to understand the person in front of us as the individual they are. But sometimes we don't and then we get caught up in games. So those games are based on how we expect that person to treat us and how we then subconsciously set up that behaviour.

'If someone in a house share is more avoidantly attached, we might notice how the games play out here too. Someone who is avoidantly attached might feel perfectly OK with having no shared space or time with their housemates. They might not seek a closeness or a connection with their housemates. Whereas someone who is insecurely attached might present to be emotionally more engaged and want more reassurance and might want attention; they might have greater relational needs from their housemates. You can find that mismatch creates confusion and misunderstanding because one doesn't understand why the other might want to spend their evening solo in their room and not in the communal space.

'It's interesting to start to notice because then you can start to say "Ah, my experience of this person might not actually be an accurate representation. This might be my projection of how I expect people to be and people to behave based on my attachment style." Ideally, then you'll seek to clarify some of those assumptions. So you can ask a housemate, "Can we just be clear what our expectations are of each other?"'

Highly attuned to others' moods and often in need of reassurance, my attachment style is at the anxious end of the spectrum. I want to feel connected to my housemates and for them to want the same, I try to avoid conflict at all costs, and find it difficult to ask for what

I need from a housemate, no matter how small that need is. The house shares where I felt I had a place are the ones where I had a calm and consistent connection with my housemates, and where, when I did need to voice an opinion or ask for something, this was met with kindness and deep understanding.

The times I have found my place in a house share – knowing the things I can contribute to the group, being empowered to make decisions, and feeling aligned with the others on how things are run – have brought a sense of purpose, calm, and clarity to my home life. Looking back on those house shares, I can see that three vital things were at play:

• the role I played in the house share complemented my personality and expectations of what home feels like
• we were all at a stage in our house sharing life cycle when the group had gelled and knew each other pretty well
• the roles had been defined and each housemate in the group was aware of and happy with the expectations placed on them.

Looking at the stages of development required to reach this sweet spot can help us to get better at actively finding our place in our house share's pecking order.

The life cycle of a house share

We're social creatures, hardwired to live in social groups. So, for decades, psychologists have been researching groups and what makes some gel and others fall apart, proposing various theories. When it comes to the different stages of development of a group, you might have heard the five-stage 'forming, storming, norming, performing, and adjourning' model. It's one that psychologists Bruce Tuckman and Mary Ann Jensen[4] created and is referenced when looking at all kinds of groups, from friendship groups to work teams.

In a house share, I think the optimum point to get to is the norming stage of group development. When you're not trying to reach a goal, just content to be living harmoniously alongside one another, this is the norming stage – the sweet spot in housemate relationships. The performing and adjourning stages aren't hugely relevant in house shares, so we won't dive into what's involved in those. Instead, we'll focus on the stages that, if we get through them, will take us to the norming stage, when people in a house share know their roles and everyone's aligned on how to behave in the space.

In the first, forming stage of a house share, though, it may feel chaotic. Like you, each housemate may have different ideas of what the house share should be. Allow some time for each of you to get acquainted with one another but, after your first month or so, it's worth opening up a conversation about how you want to approach things like cleaning the communal spaces. Spark a discussion about basic ground rules in which everyone can share something they're hoping will be respected. Then, together, you can find small ways to actively involve each member in the tasks that need to be done.

In the second, storming stage, you're likely to have established some ground rules, but there might be some conflict and tension arising over the roles and influence of each housemate. This is the most energy-sapping stage, as different personalities shine through and difficult conversations need to happen to drive the group forwards.

In the third, norming stage, you're likely to experience more of a sense of belonging and feel like you can raise problems and find solutions together without causing a huge rift in the household. Maintaining this equilibrium requires each housemate to continue voicing frustrations as they arise.

It might be that you're in a newly formed house share group, so still need to iron out some ground rules and agree on how you want to live together. It might be that you've lived there a while, but feel like you're stuck in the storming stage. Perhaps you've reached the norming stage and feel quite happy, but a new person is going to join you soon, so it would be helpful to tune in to how the group shifts when they arrive. If you're frustrated and feeling stuck in whatever stage you're in now, look at what can be done to move the group along or improve the situation. Looking back at my own house shares through the lens of group development, I can map the frustrations I felt living in them to the stage we were in as a group.

Forming

It was a wintry Sunday when I moved in to my first London house share in Elephant and Castle with Patrick, one of the five housemates living there. Even so, I'm in desperate need of a shower after breaking a serious sweat dragging a suitcase across London on two Tube lines and then two buses. I'd packed it full of things this morning, including a duvet condensed in a vacuum bag and a lamp wrapped in a towel. Now, I'm having to remind myself that it'll be worth the effort: I'll get to the house, unpack my things, make it cosy, and it'll feel more 'mine'. I got the keys earlier in the week as all five of the other housemates had plans to be out this weekend. It means I'll have some space to myself to unpack and settle in.

My room – the one I'd secured with a £700 deposit, plus £750 as my first month's rent – is a ground-floor furnished room on the right when you open the front door. I bundle in, carrying my suitcase plus a hopeful vision of what this room will be to me. But it's worse than I remembered. I'd viewed it with the rose-tinted glasses you wear when you're in need of a place to live. Now the semi-permanence of it is dawning on me – that I'll be living here for the foreseeable – I'm seeing it for the dark, cold, and drab space it is. The slatted blinds are stuck permanently ajar and the street light shines through, showing up the layers of dust that have gathered on them. I stuff the previous tenant's duvet in the wardrobe, wanting it out of the way as quickly as possible but not sure what to do with it. It feels sort of greasy and the smell's lingering on my hands. The carpet is peppered with dust, crumbs, and other signs of the life that he lived here.

I find three Hoovers[5] in various corners of the house. Not one of them works. I open the kitchen cupboards one by one, but none of them is the cleaning cupboard. I walk into the bathroom, hoping to find some cleaning things there. The sink's full of beard hair. I take a look at the shower. The plughole's barely visible under the hair that's gathered there – multiple shades, shapes, and lengths. I drop everything and walk to a supermarket to buy rubber gloves, bleach – and a Hoover.

Moving in to a new house share and discovering that the room you have to sleep in that night is filthy has to be one of the greatest disappointments on the house sharing journey. It was a sign of things to come. There was no house WhatsApp group, no kitty to buy cleaning stuff, and we each paid our rent and contribution to bills directly to the landlord. I even kept my own sponge and washing-up liquid in my room, fearing that a housemate would use the same sponge I wash my mugs with to wipe the toilet.

I can map my house share in Elephant and Castle on to Tuckman and Jensen's five-stage forming, storming, norming, performing, and adjourning model of how groups develop that we've been looking at. The chaos I experienced is symptomatic of me and my five housemates never properly forming as a group. We therefore never went on to reach the storming or norming stages.

When I look back at how the six of us functioned in the house share, we were very separate entities. I never knew who was home. For a couple of months, Patrick had a selection of friends live with us for free and the landlord had no idea. One of the other housemates, Julie, who was French, would barricade her room door shut with her wardrobe every time she went back to Paris for a weekend. She'd move the wardrobe right next to the door before slithering out of the gap she'd left, then pull the wardrobe as close to the door as she could to block the entrance to her room. All to deter Patrick from letting his mates sleep there while she was away.

Stuck in the forming stage, there was no clear idea of how we wanted our home to be. The fact that there was no structure to the group and we had no defined roles created a sense of disorder and confusion that pervaded my time living there. It manifested in awkward encounters in the communal spaces. We held stilted conversations in the kitchen when we found ourselves cooking at the same time. If I could, I'd wait until I could hear the kitchen was empty before going in there to cook. On most days, I'd see one or two of my housemates in passing, and I'd nod and smile in the hallway. We each kept our own supply of toilet paper in our bedrooms and carried a roll with us every time we needed to go. And, as well as barricading her door when she went away for the weekend, Julie kept all her food and crockery in her room, not trusting that others wouldn't take it.

In describing the first stage of a group's development, psychologists talk about the need to establish ground rules and identify roles. They also describe inhibited interactions, feelings of insecurity, and a subdued atmosphere, which summarises my experience in that house share so accurately.

The lack of clear communication between us was visibly reflected in the state of the house: we had no agreement in place as to how often and who would clean communal areas, no joint household items like a TV or Hoover, and the kitchen cupboards were managed on a find-a-space-and-fill-it basis. And sometimes, it seemed, so were the bedrooms. If something in the communal space needed doing, like the setting or disposing of mouse traps or the changing of light bulbs, it was left to whoever spotted it to sort it. Or else they assumed the next person might do it. And that's how, by the time I moved in, there'd been no working light in the downstairs toilet for as long as my housemates could remember. Leaning towers of legacy plastic food containers, discarded kitchen gadgets, and mismatched, chipped crockery filled the cupboards – a sign that tenants rotated more often than a good sort out was instigated.

Now, I can see with more clarity that our house share fell short of properly forming as a group. If I could go back in time, before accepting the room, I would have tried to initiate a conversation about how we wanted to live together and how we would work together to create an environment we were happy with. As it was, no one was motivated or interested enough in making the house share run better, so we never made it to a place where we started to see a structure develop. There were no ground rules, no sense of accountability, and no desire to take on responsibilities. We were passive bystanders in a place we called home.

Storming

It's useful knowing what the underpinnings of a functional group are when you have to run a household together, even if you're not friends with your housemates and have no desire to be. There is order and structure to how we humans behave when we are in groups as this once served to help our ancestors to fight predators and survive. When I look back at other house shares I've lived in where there have been four or five of us, I can see how this social hardwiring played out as we subconsciously moved through the stages of group development. In the second, the storming stage, there is the struggle that occurs before a pecking order is formed.

When Priya Isaacs, 31, moved into her seventh house share in Islington, north London, she picked up on the homely atmosphere and the bones of a group structure that meant tasks got done. 'It was a cosy place and the two housemates I'd be living with, a man and a woman around my age, seemed quite chilled. When we met, the woman, Thea, did most of the talking and explaining how things around the house worked. It was clear at that point she sort of ran things as she was showing me around about the flat.'

Priya's house share, more evolved than my own in Elephant and Castle, had Thea as its unofficial leader. 'When I moved in, I remember trying to find a place for some wine glasses that I had, and I moved some things out of a cupboard to make room for them. Thea wasn't very happy about that. I remember her being quite territorial, so if I moved anything, I'd consult her first. Despite that, we got on quite well for about a year and I was happy to go along with what she said. She was in charge of bills and the rent was paid through her account, so I'd transfer an amount to her each month and so would the other guy. When I wanted my blinds fixed, Thea didn't want me to get in touch with the landlord because she was worried if we asked for more that the landlord would put the rent up. She was the gatekeeper, and I had no contact with the landlord at all.

'But then Thea said we needed to pay more to cover the bills and to have some in there in case we needed back-up funds. I enquired about how much the bills were. I was aware that she was struggling with money and obviously I didn't want to make her situation worse or for her to feel like she had to move out of the house. When I looked at the bills, though, I realised I'd been overpaying for the whole time I'd lived there and I wasn't sure where the money was going. So I made a spreadsheet and explained to her I was going to pay X amount because that's what we owe and if she needs more, fine, I'll pay, but I'd like to see the bill. We just didn't see eye to eye on it. She wanted me to continue paying more and it kind of destroyed our relationship in the house. There was a time where we got on quite well but, now, whenever we're in the communal space, she puts her earphones in and I can tell I've really pissed her off because we don't see eye to eye on how the bills should be managed. There's a horrible vibe in the house.'

This sort of conflict and disagreement over roles and differences in a house share is typical of the second storming stage[6] in the group's development. It's the point when house sharers might compete, resist one another's influence, and there may be a struggle for power. I've seen this play out in the house shares I've lived in too. When everyone's finding their place, relationships take centre stage and personality types and interaction styles really come into the frame.

I remember a time this happened in the flat I shared with Phoebe, Sophie, and Jess in Balham, well before the drama with Ben. Phoebe, Sophie, and I decided to sort out the lounge, which was full of stuff left by previous housemates.

We're standing, arms folded, staring at the grotty Persian-style rug that's covering the wooden floor. We agree that it is making the room feel darker and more old-fashioned than it is. We each take a corner and roll it up, stuffing it in under the sofa. We decide that the deep-red cushions need to go, too, and squeeze them into a cupboard. We bring things down from our rooms to create a new look. Phoebe's got a beige rug and Sophie and I have some neutral-coloured cushions and throws we use to cover the stained sofas. Then we pull out the dining table that was pushed against the wall and position it so we can seat four people round it. It all feels much more sophisticated – to us. We spend hours zhuzhing it up without even thinking that we needed to consult Jess; we thought she'd be delighted.

The next day, we come home from work and find all the furniture is back how it was before, and the bits we'd brought down from our rooms are neatly folded on the corner of one of the sofas. Jess, who has been working from home, pops her head out of the door and tells us she wants to keep it this way. We should probably have discussed our plans with Jess before moving everything, but it felt as though there was a real push and pull between us all over this room rearrangement.

Some housemates can get stuck at this stage, possibly like

Priya's did, and struggle to function as a group, unable to find comfortable positions in it and move on to the next stage in the group's development.

At this point, when you're trying to establish roles and rules, politeness can keep you stuck, says Jane Sassienie, who has been coaching groups in how to be more effective in a workplace setting for more than 20 years. 'We talk about groups moving from polite positions to dialogue to cohesion. So, in a workplace, you'll see people arrive at a meeting and ask about their weekends. And in a house share, when you move in, there's lots of polite conversation, but you're probably avoiding saying what you really want. You have to, at some stage, get out of the polite phase because it usually ends up in lots of hidden things. Stuff is happening that causes anger or upset, and you can't express it; people start getting passive-aggressive. You want to get to a point where you're stating what's going on for you so you don't get stuck.

'Good conversations are really the vehicle for working together and for living together too. You have to be willing to say what is true for you, and why it's important or true for you. You don't just get stuck in your position, and then go, "No, I'm right." You question: "Why is that so important to you?" And share: "This is important to me, because…" Often, then, you have a completely new understanding of someone, and them of you.'

Norming

A few years after that Elephant and Castle house share, but before I lived with Phoebe, Jess, and Sophie, I moved into a place on Weir Road, also in Balham, where three other people had lived together for a year. I'd heard about the room through a colleague at work.

I'm in my early 20s at this point, a keen runner, and a few months into my first job on a newspaper. It's the middle of January and I'm on my way to a house party, carrier bag swinging alongside me, holding a bottle of gin, tonic, lemons, and plastic cups. I've spent three hours getting ready, sending full-length pictures of my outfits to my big sister, who told me I need to wear tights. I'm nervous because I don't know anyone going apart from my colleague, Nathalie. It's her friends who are throwing the party in the house share I'm hoping to take a room in. Knowing I was interested in the room, they extended an invite to me via Nathalie.

It's a walk from Balham Tube to where the flat is on Weir Road and, as I approach the house, I spot a few other 20-somethings carrying bags full of booze like me. I drift over, hoping Nathalie is going to be easily locatable when I get there. She's outside the front door, chatting to two guys when I arrive. I say 'Hi' and relax, knowing that I can take her lead now.

Fairy lights wrapped around the banister light the way up the stairs to the second-floor flat – the house share that could soon be mine. It's narrow, like a corridor, with the bedrooms leading off it, but a good layout for a house party. In the kitchen, halfway down the corridor, there's a big Kilner jar of punch that's drawing the attention of everyone arriving. Plastic cups and chopping boards are laid out, with knives and citrus fruit, and a huge bowl filled with ice. There are a few others making drinks, so we get chatting while slicing pieces of citrus fruit to drop into our plastic cups. I know the names of the women living here: Sima, Lottie, Margot, and Cat. It's Cat's room I'm potentially taking.

People arrive, gravitating towards the living room, at the opposite end of the flat to the kitchen. Nathalie and I follow them with our drinks. There's a group sitting down on the floor in a circle and we join it, a couple of people shuffling out to form a bigger circle so there's space for us. I get a sense of how well these people know one another and the four women who are throwing the party. I feel on the periphery of being part of something.

The evening unfolds and I get chance to chat to each of my prospective housemates and to Cat, who's moving out. Lottie shows me her rabbit, Eric, whose cage she's temporarily moved into her bedroom to protect him from the noise of the party. Cat tells me to keep an eye on how often he's being cleaned as sometimes his cage stinks but that, mostly, he's a lovely, furry addition to the flat, and he hops around when they're hanging out in the lounge. Sima just gives me a big hug and doesn't speak to me all night but, seeing how she spends the night joking and dancing, I know it was her way of saying 'Welcome'.

Two days later, I get invited to a group called Weird Road. It's the four women house sharing on Weir Road and this is all the confirmation I need to know that they'd like me to move in.

LOTTIE: Alice! Come for dinner this week and you can have a proper look at Cat's room? xx

SIMA: Yessss, we were thinking a nice cheese and wine eve on Wed? We'll all grab a diff cheese?

MARGOT: I'm cranberry Wensleydale

CAT: I'm out that eve but you guys go ahead & Alice let me know what furniture you'd like to keep once you've had a look. I'm happy to leave wardrobe/dressing table/stool but if you don't want them then I'll get rid before I go x

On moving day, Lottie makes sure I know where everything is, shows me my freezer drawer, fridge shelf, cupboard, and where the cleaning stuff is. A cleaner comes every Wednesday, she explains. She takes cash out from our joint account to leave it in a tin on the shelf for her.

I open the door to my new room and it smells like Febreze. I can see it has been hoovered.

When a new person enters a group, it does shake the group up and the development cycle starts again. As this house share group was already quite established, we moved quite quickly through the forming stage.

In the first few months, there was a bit of tension when I, the one joining the pre-existing group, expressed my specific needs and requested changes to how things were done. I was working late shifts at a newspaper at the time, so I was out in the evenings and home in the day. I had to broach the subject of putting the heating on for a couple of hours while I was working during the day.

Self-help author and coach Mike Robbins calls these 'sweaty-palmed conversations' because, however you approach them, they feel uncomfortable, but they are necessary. I was terrified to start the conversation and the therapist I was seeing at the time got me to practise using 'I statements'. The idea of these is that all you do is share your own feelings on something and allow the other person to respond. So instead of saying something like, 'It's really unfair I'm paying for heating I won't be there to feel the benefit of, so you should amend the heating times', I'd make it about me. I often typed it out in the Notes app on my phone first to try it out:

'I'd like to switch the heating on for an hour longer in the morning and earlier in the evening so that I can keep warm when I'm at home in the daytime.'

'I feel worried about being cold when I'm at home in the daytime before I start my shift, and I'd like to put the heating on for an extra hour in the morning and the evening.'

In response, the others raised concerns about the cost. We decided we'd give it a trial run, to see if it was really expensive, then worked out timings that we were all happy with.

Research shows that, in the window after entering a group, new-comers do have the influence to bring about changes.[8] In a house share setting, then, shortly after moving in is a good time to request a change or suggest things that would work better for you – a kitchen cupboard of your own, perhaps, or getting a working Hoover between you.

The year that followed was a sociable one. As a house share group, we tended to Eric the rabbit, committed to 'flat-sorting mornings', when we'd spend a Saturday morning each month sprucing the place up. We threw more parties and came together for cheese and wine nights, and house roasts. Conflicts arose – mostly sparked by a message in the house WhatsApp group – but we were motivated to get things back on track.

The structure and order in place in that house share meant we were each free to enjoy the rest of our time there. My more settled experience hit the sweet spot in the stages of group development and so chimes with the definition of the norming stage. This, typically, is a point when the behaviour of those in the group is more alike than in earlier stages, but there are clear differences between the position and purpose each individual has in the group. A state of equilibrium is reached regarding tasks and social aspects – the group is in a comfortable space where everyone knows their place.[9] I see now that this happened because there was a clear leader in Lottie, while Sima came a close second, and Margot and I were happy to conform. The delineation and hierarchy of our roles, though unspoken, created a homely atmosphere in the house share.

In the Weir Road house share, then, there was a structure, an order, and a clear place for me. 'Cohesion is a state of having done the hard work,' explains Jane. 'You get to this kind of good, balanced place, and everybody knows what everyone needs. You make moves that are right for each other. You're not just moving on your own behalf.'

It takes work to get to this point of equilibrium, and maintaining this state requires constant reassessment as tenancies change and house share groups form and re-form. 'When someone new joins, the whole group is thrown up in the air and you're sort of starting again,' says Jane.

At the helm of the house share

The transition of moving in to the Weir Road flat and the process leading to me feeling at home was much easier than in previous moves because Lottie was an unofficial leader figure, bringing order and much needed clarity. She had somehow landed the responsibility of being the bill keeper and, as a result, people treated and regarded her as the leader in the house.

It does tend to be the person who was in the house share first who takes on the leadership role. That's what happened in this case, with Lottie and Sima explaining to me how things were done when I moved in. And when Priya joined her Islington house share with Thea, there was already an established hierarchy.

Olivia Lock is 32 and in her eighth house share in Oxford. She lives with three other women, but she's been in the house the longest. Having lived in other house shares where the responsibility for bills was shared, she thinks that having one person at the helm is the best set-up.

'I do all the bills and it kind of falls on me to be the one who's responsible for everything,' she says. 'I lived in a flat before where each one of us had responsibility for a bill and I just didn't think it worked. It got really confusing, with transferring money over and stuff, so I took it over here when a previous tenant moved out. I've made sure everyone in this house is on a bill, so they've got something for ID checks and the like, and we're all on the council tax, but it all comes out of one account. And then we've just got a bank card, which, if we need anything for the house, the girls can take the bank card away. I've subscribed us to a few things, like monthly toilet roll deliveries, because I don't want the responsibility to follow me to pick these things up. I've got a Google doc sheet, which has got all the passwords for every single bill and everything, that I've shared with the house. I update it but everyone has access to it.

'I have to have those awkward conversations, like, "Guys, the heating cost has gone up, so the bills are going to go up and this is what it's going to cost." Then I have to check I'm actually getting the money. And then, if we've got a surplus, I'll need to ask them what they want to do with it – transfer it or do we go out as a house for food or drinks? In terms of mental load and stuff, I find it's a lot more than if you lived on your own.'

What Olivia describes is backed up by research, which suggests that, in a group setting, if you appear more task-orientated than the others in the group, you are perceived as having more influence,[10] and the same is true if you talk more than your fellow members; 'I don't like saying it, but I do feel that I'm the one in charge.'

Also, as Olivia has outlined, if someone's taking charge of the money side, they need to be transparent about how they're managing it. Even if someone is simply organising the cleaning rota and who buys what, there needs to be a central place where the others can access information about where their money is going. Research into leadership in the workplace shows that, when leaders behave with transparency, communicating the rationale behind their decisions, this has a positive impact on the psychological safety of those they are leading, resulting in attention and creativity.[11] It makes sense that this also applies in a house share situation, as we feel safer when we are given insights into how decisions are made and where our money is going.

Like Priya, living in a house share in Islington where she had a disagreement with her housemate about the bills, I had a tricky situation arise in one of my house shares, where I lived with three others. I found out that the housemate in charge of the rent had upped my rent to knock rent off their own room, despite their room being twice the size of mine. I'd agreed to take my room at a fixed price when I moved in, assuming that my housemate's rent would be fixed by the landlord at a higher level because it's bigger than mine. But I discovered later, after seeing a document from the landlord, that, because my housemate was gathering rent from all of us to make one payment to the landlord each month, she had fixed her own rent at a lower level and put mine up to cover some of her share. I was unknowingly paying a portion of her rent. When I found out she was mismanaging the money, I lost a lot of trust in her. I never brought it up because I was due to move out a few months later and I had agreed to the price of the room on moving in. But I now know that needing to be cautious about how money is being managed where you are living makes it hard to feel at home.

'In the work I do with teams in the workplace, we often talk about there being multiple hierarchies,' says Jane. 'There are the people who got there first, but then there's the positional hierarchy of job role, which might not be the same as the people who got there first. You do kind of get more organised when there's a leader. But it's never as easy as saying "You're the leader", and that's the end of it because the roles in groups are always contextual.' So in a house share, you've got the person who got there first, the person who's taking the lead on the bills, the person who spends most time there.

Looking at the stage your own house share has reached in terms of developing as a group can be empowering. You may be able to see some necessary tweaks that would benefit your group of housemates and make you feel more at home. Overlaying this with the role you played in your home growing up, your own attachment style, and how that shapes your ideas of what home feels like can help to join the dots of an otherwise chaotic organisational structure. Mapping the other roles you've played in groups throughout your life as well can really inform your decisions, so you can either choose the type of house share set-up you want to move in to or retro-engineer the one you're in, so it works well with your personal blueprint of the role you play in a group.

Chapter reflections

Can you reflect on your upbringing, the family hierarchies, and how they've shaped what home looks and feels like?

When you look at your own family when you were growing up, can you see how it's shaped the role that you're naturally drawn to or enjoy playing most in your friendship groups? Perhaps you can use this to inform what you're looking for in a house share and think about making the role you play in your house share work to your strengths and what feels familiar and homely to you.

Can you draw the rough organisational structure of your house share, showing the different hierarchies at play?

Who arrived first? Who spends most time there? Who sorts out the bills? Does someone have more ownership of the space than the others? All these hierarchies are active beneath the surface of your interactions. Identifying them and acknowledging them is helpful in understanding one another.

How can you bring your housemates together to strengthen how you make decisions and operate as a group?

Think about the different stages outlined in this chapter to work out which one your house share is in at the moment. Are there ways in which you think you or your housemates would benefit from becoming a more cohesive group? How might you be able to work towards making these things happen?

Can you practise having a sweaty-palmed conversation about something that might disrupt the current pecking order in your house share?

Perhaps you've just moved in and it seems the other housemates don't routinely take the bins out, but this is something that's important to you. You can choose anything, from something small that feels like it's not worth bringing up – such as not picking up the bath mat – or something bigger – like you're not happy about how often your housemate's boyfriend is coming over.

Whether your conversation will disrupt the hierarchy based on who was there first, who spends most time there, or who has most responsibility for the space, think about which one of these makes your request feel challenging. Without filtering anything out, how do you feel about it? Can you tell a friend about the thing and vent via a voice note?

Now try to create a filtered version, using 'I statements' that you could genuinely say to your housemate to share your feelings and allow your housemate to respond. This means, instead of saying, 'I need you to pull your weight and clean the bathroom because I've done it every week for two months', you would make it about you: 'I've got loads on my plate at the moment and not being able to find the time to clean the bathroom properly is really stressing me out.' Try typing them out in your Notes app to check what wording works best.

6. Rental Health

Managing mental wellbeing in a house share

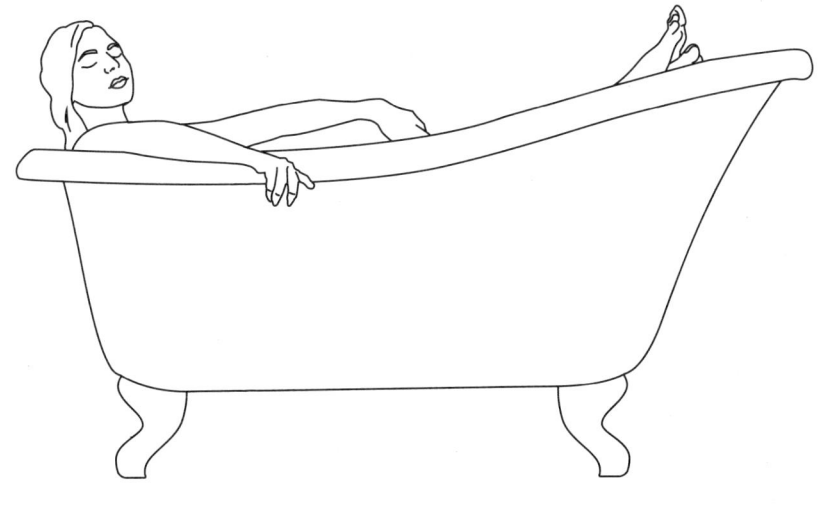

"Accept thoughts, but don't become them…
You can walk through a storm and feel the
wind, but you know you are not the wind"

Matt Haig[1]

While one hand is lying flat on my stomach, the other is resting on my chest, over my heart. I count my breaths silently, following what the Headspace app says: in 1–2–3–4, hold 1–2–3–4, out 1–2–3–4.

I'm in my room in the house share in Elephant and Castle, where I lived with five others, and I'm trying very hard to tune in to the floor that's supporting the bed and me, telling myself that I am safe. I note that I am surrounded by my familiar things, the stuff I brought here to make the room feel like home. The lamp, the print on the wall, the clothes draped over the chair. I breathe in the familiar scent of my washing powder on the sheets. But it's gone 1am on a Tuesday and I've woken up to the front door opening and footsteps of three, possibly four, people walking into the house. My room is right by the hall and, in the stillness and dark, the sounds of these people kicking off their shoes and their coats brushing against my door feels invasive.

I'm stuck in a cycle that you might know all too well: my mind is telling me that this is my room, my house share, but my body is tense and I don't feel like I'm at home.

I can make out my housemate's voice, but there are two or three other voices that I don't recognise. I don't know whether it's because there are strangers in my home or there's no lock on my door, but I feel on edge. Maybe it's because they're about to keep me up all night. And it would be perfectly reasonable for these people to assume that the door to the room on the ground floor – my room – is the bathroom and so come in unannounced. My body feels sort of frozen now and I'm staring into the darkness, reminding myself that it is normal and OK for my housemate to have friends over. But feeling as though you have little or no control over your home environment has an impact on your mental health.

Peeling back the layers

When there's a push and pull between your needs and your housemates' needs, and it's happening in real time, 24/7, in your home, it leads to a unique type of low-level but continual anxious rumination that I'm going to call 'house share hypervigilance'. It's a pervasive heightened state of awareness of your environment and the people around you. This is something other people expect when they go on holiday or visit a new city, but this is happening in your home, all the time. While comic horror stories from house shares make the headlines, the toll that the ever-present friction of dealing with and considering others in your personal space takes on your mental health doesn't attract the same level of attention. And yet, for the majority of house sharers, this is the all-encompassing reality of daily life.

Nearly half (41–47 per cent) of 16–39-year-olds responding to a survey in the UK in 2024 said they feel anxious or stressed all or most of the time.[2] In the USA, in 2023, more than half of 16–39-year-olds reported that they had gone or were currently going to therapy, with 76 per cent of them citing anxiety as the reason.[3] Anxiety stems from more than just one cause but, for me, the politics and temporary nature of house sharing certainly don't help. It's no coincidence that the year I took medication for anxiety – at a loss as to how else I could calm my cripplingly busy mind – was the year I was living in Elephant and Castle. It was one of the most stressful house shares I have experienced.

There are layers on layers of anxiety-inducing factors at play when you're living in a house share. On the surface, there are housemate politics, cleaning rotas, and bills. Then there's the fact that your physical space is not your own and you have to contend with housemates' lifestyles which, as we've seen, don't always complement yours. There's also the impact that this incompatibility can have on how you feel about yourself. Plus, there's the lack of control that comes from relying on a landlord to replace the washing machine if it breaks down or – as happened in one of my house shares – to deal with a pigeon infestation. It's estimated that almost a quarter – 23 per cent – of occupied private rented-sector dwellings in the UK fail the Decent Homes Standard,[4] leaving house sharers in run-down spaces, dealing with dripping taps and damp.

Beneath all these layers, there is the impermanence of the whole situation, which I think is key. At any point, your rental contract could be terminated or a housemate might decide to move on, changing the dynamics of the house share. A survey of 834 young, single adults living in Seoul, South Korea,[5] highlighted three main areas that weigh on the mental health of house sharers. First, the lack of control over circumstances and housemates. Second, negative feelings about house sharing and what it says about your identity. And, third, a lack of stability.

When you think about it, it's not surprising that renters are twice as likely to experience anxiety as homeowners.[6] And, while there's an alarming lack of statistics outlining the impact of house shares on mental health considering how many of us actually live in them, each piece of research that has been done draws the same conclusion: because of the quality of the housing and other people's behaviour, living in house shares is linked to poor mental health.[7]

And, for me, the inner voice that accompanies this low-level stress, even after years of house sharing, goes something like this: 'Did I wash up my plates or did they wash them? Are they trying to make a point? Has someone been using my olive oil? I swear I had a whole bottle, but I can't be sure. I'd like to have a bath now but are my housemates going to get home from work and need the toilet? I've been in the bath 30 minutes, I'd better get out so they don't get pissed off. Am I entitled to be annoyed that they woke me up last night? Yes, I am. No, I'm not. I'll say something. No, I won't. I've said something. Maybe I shouldn't have. Are they still going to like me? Someone's definitely been using my olive oil. I'll send a text to ask. Or maybe that's passive-aggressive. I'll ask later…' And so the continual self-questioning and monitoring of my home environment and the relationships in it continues.

Back to the early hours of that Tuesday morning when I was woken up by Patrick and his mates piling in through the front door. I'm still lying on my bed and, through the soothing sound of the Headspace instructions, I can hear them moving into the kitchen. I get up and stuff a towel in the gap under my door. I'd be embarrassed if they heard me doing that – a woman in her 20s behaving like a child, afraid of monsters under her bed.

An hour later, I wake again to the group in the kitchen laughing loudly. I'm lying there, paralysed by indecision. Is this my problem? Am I too uptight? Or is it reasonable for me to ask them to go somewhere else? It's a work night and I need to sleep.

The logical answer is to go and ask them to be quiet. But I'm trapped in a perpetual cycle of being angry that my housemates aren't more considerate and worrying that I'm being unreasonable and that this is a me problem. I am, after all, a 20-something in a house share where YOLO is the code of conduct.

I get out of bed, pull a jumper on, take a deep breath, push the door open, and walk into the kitchen. Their conversation stops and everyone's eyes are on me.

'Hey.' I give them a forced smile, deliberately squinting my eyes to make the point that I've just woken up. 'Do you guys mind just keeping it down a bit? I've got to be in the office really early tomorrow.'

Patrick apologises immediately and begins ushering his friends out the door. I shuffle back to my room, feeling heartened by his response but worried that he might be pissed off. My body, though, feels the relief. I climb back into bed, calmer.

Tiny traumas

On a very physical level, continually censoring your own behaviour and monitoring your environment triggers a 'fight or flight' response in your body, as do small passive-aggressive comments from housemates, and frustrations over money and cleanliness. The cumulative effect of these micro-stresses has, in the past, left me heading towards emotional burnout. Because, when you're dealing with these subtle but never-ending daily stresses in your own home, you have little physical space or mental distance available to you so you can recover from the stress response that's occurring in your body.

These small, seemingly insignificant daily frustrations are the types of 'psychological scrapes' that inspired psychologist Dr Meg Arroll's book, *Tiny Traumas*.[8] I ask her for her insights into how, over time, these small irritations can wear away at our mental wellbeing. 'The damaging thing about tiny traumas – and I know from my own years living in a house share there are many that can arise – is that they're repetitive. When something irritates you, you might think at the time "Oh, that's not a big deal", but those small things build up and build up,' Meg says.

Eve Watson, 28, is a teacher and has been house sharing in Liverpool for three years. She, too, finds herself stuck in unhelpful cycles of feeling irritated and then doubting herself. Eve describes a recent incident: 'I've got a draining rack and the other day someone put stuff on there that wasn't properly washed, and I was really annoyed about it because it was making my stuff dirty, so I moved all their stuff off it and put the rack away before I went to work. And I knew it would be really obvious what I'd done. But then, all day at work, I was like, was that too passive-aggressive? Should I have done that?'

Part of what makes these tiny traumas so insidious is that they're the small things we often dismiss because we don't feel we have the right to complain about them. 'If you don't address what's going on, especially in your home, it might start to have an impact on your behaviour and how you feel about yourself,' says Meg.

Eve describes exactly that happening, these small irritations leaving her questioning herself all the time. 'You do have these weird, intrusive thoughts where you think it's all you,' she says. 'The number of times I lie in bed at night and think to myself, "Is it me? Is that why I can't live with anyone?" And then it spirals and I start thinking – "Am I actually impossible to live with?"'

Letting these tiny traumas go unnoticed and not acknowledging them means that we can end up turning in on ourselves and starting to think it's a me problem. 'Humans are meaning-making machines,' says Meg. 'We will always try to make meaning out of whatever situation we're in. So if we feel low as a result of an accumulation of small things that have been annoying in the house share and it's not obvious why and we can't find a reason or an explanation, then we blame ourselves. We tell ourselves it must be us, that we're oversensitive, or not resilient enough, or not good at communicating. When we don't have a framework and we don't understand tiny traumas and how they build up, we will internalise them and start to think it's us, our fault. So looking at these tiny traumas and giving them space helps our brains understand that it's not us, it's the situation.'

She continues, 'I've been asked so many times, "How do we avoid them, these tiny traumas?" But we don't; they happen all the time. It's not about avoiding them, it's about using the experience to build up our psychological immune system, and to see them as emotional antibodies. When we take all those experiences we've had and show ourselves that we can deal with them, what we have at the end of the day is this massive psychological toolkit.

'It's so important to recognise tiny traumas as they arise. And to be very, very self-compassionate when they do. We tend to do what I call reverse misery trumps. So we'll say to ourselves, "Actually, something worse happened to someone else, so I shouldn't be getting annoyed that my housemate hasn't washed up." But those two things can exist at the same time. That terrible thing could have happened to someone else and the tiny trauma can still be happening to you right now. Both things exist. They both warrant validation and recognition, and giving those tiny traumas room so we can deal with them will mean we can move forwards to really thrive.

'By unpicking some of the tiny traumas and thinking, "Oh, actually, you know, there are some of these things I can do something about" – and it may not be all of them, but there will be some – we build up that perceived control muscle again and you start thinking, "OK, I do have influence over my life."'

In her book, Meg outlines her method for doing this: her 'AAA approach'. This stands for awareness, acceptance, and action. Awareness is the first step, which is noticing what things irritate you and how they're affecting your life. Acceptance, the next step, is acknowledging that they are having an influence on your life. 'This is the stage I see many people try to piggy-back over,' says Meg, explaining that accepting how these sometimes very small things have an impact on you is the most challenging part of the process. The third step in Meg's AAA approach is action – taking steps to remedy the tiny traumas and improve things.

Writing these traumas down is a good place to start, to help your brain to process what's happening. 'You'll begin to build up a bit of a diary,' she says. 'So when you start feeling a difficult emotion – frustration or anger – sit down and try to identify what is going on. Who is there? What are they doing that's making you feel like that?' By collecting that information, you'll start to see patterns appear and notice that some of it might be external, to do with your housemate's behaviour or your house share, and some will be to do with what's going on for you.

Meg describes how being a light sleeper, like me, was the source of lots of tiny traumas when she house shared. 'I had to work to accept that was part of who I was,' she says. 'My action, then, was to be clear about my needs to my other housemates and take measures to protect my sleep. It's about learning to work *with* ourselves, not *against* ourselves. If we don't do that, over time, the accumulation of these tiny traumas can result in a constant undercurrent of melancholy and niggling anxiety.'

Shallow roots

When you feel out of control of your living space, it's sometimes easiest to disconnect from the house share. You might fall into just regarding it as a place where you sleep rather than face up to the things that you want to change to make it feel like home.

Eve explained that she does this, creating a mental distance between where she lives and her idea of 'home'. She says, 'I wouldn't call my house share "home", even though I spend the majority of my life here. A lot of my frustrations in the house are with cleanliness, but I've actually never been in a house share where I've had a conversation about it because I just don't see the point. It's not a permanent place. I just get silently annoyed and try to calm myself down by telling myself it's not for ever. I think I distance myself from the space as much as possible to cope, but then I find it really depressing that I'm in my late 20s and don't really have a place that I want to call home.'

Psychotherapist Alex Iga Golabek, runs a practice called Ego Therapy, where she works with clients to build emotional strength through focussing on acceptance. I ask for her insights into why we might disassociate (when we disconnect from our thoughts and might feel a bit detached from what's happening around us) and whether creating that distance is something we subconsciously do to create emotional distance from things that irritate us while living in a house share. 'We disassociate because of a perceived threat,' she says. 'When we feel afraid, disassociation is a very powerful tool. It's one we learn as children because we're so vulnerable and we have no other means of power or control. As a child, the only way that we can control what's happening to us, and how we are experiencing it, is by disassociation. The mind's protecting us from the impact of painful experiences we aren't equipped to handle. So we learn it as kids and then it comes with us as a tool into adulthood.

'In a house share situation, I can see how, on the one hand, it has protective qualities because it's stopping the impact of what's happening in the immediate environment – the frustrations and things we can't control – from touching us. But, on the other hand, when you disassociate, you're not allowing yourself to connect to the people or the place, which does have an impact on how you feel about yourself, your identity, and your mental wellbeing. The very thing that's protecting you is also the thing that's preventing you from calling a space home. Trying to be protected is not a bad thing – we all want to feel safe – but there's probably some work to be done to find a middle ground where you're protecting yourself enough but not preventing yourself from connection.'

I've created distance myself in house shares when things haven't been going well. I've spent more time at work or gone to stay with family or friends at weekends. I couldn't always articulate what the one thing was that made me not want to be there – it was just a general sense of feeling exhausted by the continual compromising required.

Having a fixed address and a permanent home to live in for the foreseeable future is an ideal that I've carried with me from a young age. I know that my own preconceptions of what I thought a home should look like – a two-up two-down where I'd be living with a husband by 25 – haunted me a lot for the first few years I was house sharing. Not challenging those ideals meant I looked at my house sharing life through a lens that always left me disappointed with where I was in my life. Instead of accepting, finding connection, and enjoying it, I would fixate on the fact that it wasn't where I wanted to be. So I created distance from it and continued to remind myself that it was temporary, and behaving as though it were temporary became my coping mechanism.

Eve has the same ideals weighing on her. 'I can't help but remember those pictures in primary school I drew of my future self, and I would always draw myself with a nice house and a cat or a dog. And then I look at my actual life and I don't even have a box to put my name to. In the day to day, I do just muddle through. I'm fine – it's not like I'm being hurt – but it is a depressing thought to me that I might be house sharing for ever.'

I ask Alex how we might be able to remedy these feelings of disappointment that we're not where we imagined we'd be and allow ourselves to connect to our homes, even if they don't look like the ones we'd perhaps imagined for ourselves. She says, 'Look at expectations that you bring with you. We have an unconscious drive to recreate the familiar – what we grew up with or societal norms. To what degree are you trying to recreate the familiar in a way that's helping you? And to what degree are you doing that in a way that's harmful? It's not your fault that the housing market is difficult. You can't change that. It's terrible, but there's nothing you can do about the fact you live in a generation that's faced with these systemic issues. We can't fight gravity. Are you going to be pissed off at gravity? When you accept gravity exists, you can, instead, put your energy into finding a path that works with it. Perfection doesn't exist wherever you live. So, ask yourself, in the living situation you're in, what will be good enough?'

As well as reframing what a 'good enough' home looks like, distinguishing between real and perceived threats is a powerful way to stay connected to the house shares we live in.

I think about my reaction to my housemate waking me up that night when I lived in Elephant and Castle. I knew it wasn't a real threat, but as a perceived threat, it was enough to send me into an anxious spin. I had to coach my body through the fear I felt in that moment and prove to myself I wasn't in any real danger.

'The older we get, the more experiences we have, the more fear we will have. That's natural,' says Alex. 'You're not being paranoid because these perceived threats are usually based on things that have happened to you – you were kept up all night once and it meant you couldn't go to work. Fear is part of you and it's a mechanism that has good intentions to protect you. It does go overboard and then it's down to you to befriend it and say, "Thanks, but I don't need you right now." In time, that part of you will calm down.

'You can do some experimentation on your own to see whether the threat is actually there. Look around your room and ask yourself, are you safe? Is there any real danger? Is it really the case that if you tell your housemates you'd like things to be cleaner, they wouldn't listen? Is it really the case that you can't make tweaks that would make you feel like you can call the house share "home"? Would chatting to the housemates more make it feel more like home? Put these perceived threats to the test. And see whether you're able to feel connection to the place and to the others living there.'

By experimenting in these ways and interrogating whether these are real or perceived threats, you're stopping yourself from disconnecting completely and, instead, integrating yourself into the space and the house share. It may come with frustrations and niggles but also connection.

Cora Mills, 26, is a social worker and has been living in her first house share in Hackney for three years. She's found that, by investing in the space and her housemates, she's learned to be braver about asserting her needs. As a result, she thinks that living in a house share has soothed her anxiety.

'I'd been living in the house share for a couple of months before I was diagnosed with anxiety. Ever since I told them, they've been amazing. They're so kind. Sometimes I'll leave the house and I'll be like, "Oh my God, did I turn my straighteners off?" or "Did I leave the oven on?" I'll be worried sick about it and so they'll check and reassure me. It happens all the time. Tom, who I live with, he'll make sure every evening that the back door is locked for me because I find it really hard to sleep at night. So Tom, every night, goes and checks it for me and I don't worry about it. Little things like that I'd find really tricky if I was on my own. I'd be waking up in the night and wanting to check the door's shut or I'd get to work and need to come home to check something's off.

'I have people-pleasing tendencies, which can be hard in a house share because I'm constantly checking, "Is this OK? Is this the right way? Can we try it this way? Am I doing this and this right?" It can be quite tiring. I live with two others and one of them is really direct and it works really well. He says it how it is, which I love because I'm like, "OK, you're not going to be secretly annoyed with me about something" because I know he'll tell me if he's annoyed. If I've had people over and I've been up late and had too much to drink in the lounge, I know it's a bit annoying for him because it'll have kept him up, because his room's above. Then, the next day I'll say, "I'm really sorry" and he's like, "No, don't worry about it, you never keep me up." But then, even the next day, I'm still worrying, so I'll say, "I'm still worried I've upset you" and it's quite nice that he can reassure me. I like having that communication, so things don't just fester. If he wasn't so easy to communicate with, it would be hard for me because I'd be too nervous to say something.'

In these small but significant ways, Cora integrated herself into her house share. By checking out what were real threats and what were merely perceived ones, and having conversations with her housemates to work with her to make things better, she connected to the house share and it's somewhere she now calls home.

Points of connection

The connections we form with our housemates have the power to make a hugely positive impact on our mental wellbeing. 'People are very important to feeling connected to a place,' says psychotherapist Alex. 'And human connection is very important to our health – mental and physical. The people you live with are a resource.'

Looking at your social connections as a whole and where your housemates sit within those can help you to reflect on the expectations you have of your house share. It might be that you have a fulfilling career and you're very close to your colleagues, you have a friendship group you see often, or you spend lots of time with your family. If you're feeling well connected elsewhere in your life, it's likely going to be easier to view your connections with your housemates to be of a lighter kind. On the flip side, if your house share, for now, is the place where you are getting the majority of your social connections from, then perhaps it's a space you will benefit from investing in and putting your energy into.

It might be that your housemate connections are serving you well right now, as you've moved cities and jobs, so you feel at peace with the impermanence and pour your energy into understanding some of the tiny traumas. It might be that the impermanence is serving you right now because you're hoping to change jobs or move cities, so you make peace with the daily tiny traumas and pour your energy into the connections with your housemates. It might be that you're at a place where you've worked on the tiny traumas and pour your energy into understanding some of the feelings of impermanence.

Four years have passed since I lived with Patrick and co. in Elephant and Castle and I'm living in the flat on Weir Road with Lottie and Sima. I wake to the two of them getting home from a night out. It's around midnight on Thursday and I'm doing early shifts at the newsroom this week, meaning I have to get up at 5am the next morning. The door to my room has a huge glass panel in it, so when they switch the light on in the kitchen, it shines through. I hear them whispering and quickly shuffling around the kitchen, making food and tea. Then, after a couple of minutes, the light goes off, and I hear them tiptoeing to their rooms. They know I'm on earlies that week because I've moaned about it enough times. They care and that, I learned, is what I need from a house share.

I felt calmest in the house shares where I connected with the people, was comfortable enough to share what I needed to feel at home, and committed to making each one a place we all wanted to be. The frustrations over cleanliness and the impermanence still occurred, but when I felt like my housemates were on my side, we were dealing with them together.

When I look back on the eight house shares I've lived in and the connections I made, I see how they brought a lot of joy, fun, and company to my life, outweighing some of the more frustrating aspects of house sharing.

In a society where around half 16–39-year-olds report regularly feeling lonely,[9] the social connections possible in house shares offer a solution. That is the experience of Sian Foster, a 36-year-old writer living in Glasgow, who is house sharing for the first time since separating from the partner she lived with for 18 years. 'After living alone for a little while and then travelling alone, I learned that living alone was more detrimental to my mental health,' she says.

'I'm self-employed and I work from home, so it's quite easy to slip into not prioritising my self-care. I'd wake up and work in my pyjamas until the afternoon. When you live alone, there's nobody there to hold you accountable. I live in a house share now with one other woman and respecting the other person I live with encourages me to respect the space and respect myself, so I'll clean more and I'll make sure my dishes are done. I just take better care of myself when there's someone else there to witness how I'm living.'

But while the presence of Sian's housemate is a positive for her, their relationship is very functional. She appreciates another person being there, but the level of connection is very light. 'For me, not knowing my housemate has been really, really good. It means I can come home and have a brief chat, but we live our own separate lives. She works in an office and I work from home, we don't really socialise, and it's been really nice not to have that added layer of maintaining a friendship. Having a degree of separation means I get my own privacy and space.'

Sian also speaks positively about the impermanence her house share offers. 'I'm definitely in that kind of transitional phase of where I'm like, "Oh, I thought my life was going to be this way and I thought the future was going to unfold in a certain way." And now, it's uncertain, but I'm trying to see that as a positive, and having a temporary living situation allows me to look at travelling or have flexibility to get up and go if I decide I want to. Even though our perceived lack of independence is what puts us into house shares, most people probably do have a degree of freedom and independence that perhaps you don't have when you live with a partner or with family. Because you can kind of come and go and do whatever you please in your space. You do have to consider other people, but not to the same degree as when you're in a relationship or living with family.'

For both Cora and Sian, their housemates are a source of feelings of connection that have a positive impact on their mental health because they suit what they need from their housemates. Two communication psychologists, Jeffrey Hall and Andy Merolla, looked at the patterns of people's daily social interactions to see the impacts they had on their quality of life. Their research showed that 'interaction choice' was a key factor in whether socialising improved people's wellbeing. They noticed that people who were instigators, deciding how and when their social interactions took place, reaped the benefits of social connections more than those who waited to be invited or whose interactions were incidental rather than the result of making a choice.

So, choosing how and when to connect with your housemates, as Sian and Cora have, is key. But it's not always easy. Striking the right balance between connection and privacy in a house share requires continual recalibration and serious boundary setting.

The stress contagion

I'm thinking back to when I was living in my house share in Balham with Phoebe, Jess, and Sophie, and Jess has been going through a nasty situation at work. Just home from work myself, I'm making a cup of tea in the kitchen when she gets in. I sense it's been another bad day as she's walking up the stairs to our second-floor flat while ranting down the phone to her mum. She sits down and I make her a tea, then sit opposite her trying, with the limited knowledge I have of her workplace politics, to listen and offer support. But it is the third evening this week that's been spent like this and, while I'm wanting to offer my support, inside, my own work stress is building up: I have a piece of writing waiting for me that I need to finish for a deadline tomorrow.

This has been going on for a few weeks at this point – Jess coming home and offloading her work stresses on me, almost immediately, without checking whether I'm in a place to listen to them or have other stuff to get on with. Sometimes there are tears, but, other times, she's wound up and angry, and, though she isn't shouting at me, when she raises her voice, I can feel my own stress levels rising.

I'm working long hours and trying very hard to keep my own inner calm – doing lots of yoga and breathing exercises – and really struggling to handle her work problems as well as my own. I don't want to be rude or unkind or act like I don't care – I do care – but I need my own space and time to recuperate.

In a house share, it's virtually impossible to carve out space and time, and be transparent about when you're in a communal space to socialise, support, or listen, and when you're not. In the end, I avoided being in the kitchen when Jess got home from work and, before long, though it went against every bone in my body, I stopped asking her how her day had been.

I wish I'd had some sort of card like they give you in yoga that says, 'Yes, I'm open to adjustments' or, 'No, thank you', so that housemates could be honest about what they are able to take on. Unfortunately, the only way to strike this balance is to say either, 'I'm really sorry, but I don't have the capacity to listen to this' – which, to me, feels really unkind – or to avoid the space they're in. My therapist at the time suggested that, when I entered a space Jess was in and she started talking to me about things I couldn't take on, I should imagine a shield around me – a 'protection barrier' that her problems couldn't penetrate, even though I was listening to her. That way I could preserve my energy levels and be clear about when I needed to leave the room.

In theory, it is an easy solution, but it takes a fair amount of mental energy to execute. I'd take a deep breath before I walked into the conversation and be continually reminding myself not to absorb the stress. I'd let her say what she needed to say, respond lightly, then try to communicate that I had things I needed to focus on that evening. I'd say something like, 'Oh, I'm sorry you had a rubbish day. Mine was tiring, too. I'm actually just going to make this tea and go and read my book.'

So perhaps the key to making house sharing work *with* your mental wellbeing rather than against it lies in knowing your own needs and interrogating the role your housemates play in your life. Once you know what you need from your house share, you can begin to ask for it and implement the boundaries that help you to strike a balance between mental space and connection. Then, you can really begin to invest in the people and place to make it a good enough home for now, and nurture your mental health and wellbeing.

Chapter reflections
What does a 'good enough' home look like to you?
I think we all have an image of those picture-perfect houses we drew as children. Knowing what you know now and with the

housing market as it is, if house sharing is where you're at for the foreseeable future, how can you make sure it's good enough? Somewhere that isn't perfect but meets your needs to a degree that's easy enough to live with. Being realistic, what are the things you can look for and ask for that allow you to exercise a level of control over your living situation?

Ask, 'What's working for me here and what isn't?'
At any one time, there needs to be a factor in your house share that is working for you, makes the other aspects more bearable, and gives you the energy you need to work on making one aspect better. Framing it like this can help you to settle on what 'good enough' looks like while you're working on the aspects that aren't yet good enough. Somewhere on the spectrum between perfect and intolerable is good enough. This is where our non-negotiables and basic needs are being met, but we may need to compromise on other preferences. There might be some factors that need to be put to one side while you focus on one that's more important or affects your mental wellbeing the most. Of the three factors – tiny daily traumas, the impermanence of your living situation, and your connections in the house share – is there:

- one that is serving you
- one that you can make peace with
- one that you could pour more energy into?

How can you stay grounded?
Practising one of the various grounding techniques is a simple but powerful way to anchor yourself in a space if you're feeling fear, a threat, or a tiny trauma. What are the activities that allow you to take a moment to tune in to whether the threat you're facing is perceived or real? Maybe you already practise mindfulness or have a calming breathing technique that helps you. Alex suggests trying this simple

grounding technique in the first instance. 'Look around your room. Are you safe? Is there danger? Is there a threat? Remind yourself that you're not in immediate danger. This should be your starting point.'

In moments of high stress, go back to basics
'It can be really easy to forget about the things that regulate our emotional, physical, and mental health,' says psychologist Meg. 'But these can help lift your mood enough to face up to difficult conversations or take action towards improving your situation. Go back to basics. Think about small steps that will nurture your physical health. Sleep, move, get out in nature. When we're in a heightened state and a stressful environment, these things tend to go out the window. Go back and focus on them.'

How can you make room to process your tiny traumas or perceived threats more constructively?
Next time something small gets your back up and you feel yourself getting even a little bit stressed, acknowledge that it's a tiny trauma and give yourself the time and headspace to think about what's happening. If you can, write out a tiny trauma using Meg's AAA approach described earlier in this chapter: awareness, acceptance, action. The first step (awareness) is writing down what irritates you and how it's affecting your life. The second step (acceptance) is trying to be at peace with the fact that it's having an impact on your life. The final step (action) is thinking about what you could do to resolve it – asking your housemate not to do something that's irritating you, for example.

Can you carry out a reality check?
'When you're dealing with a tiny trauma and there are others involved, it is really common to attempt some mind reading,' says Meg. 'So, instead of having a conversation with a person, you might start to assume that you know what the other person is thinking.' It's natural to project experiences that we've had growing

up and in early relationships on to situations we find ourselves in as adults, but sometimes this can lead us to make unhelpful assumptions about a person or a situation. 'Stop yourself and challenge some of those thoughts,' continues Meg. 'Ask, "Is this accurate? Is this sensible? Is this kind?" It's a good way of breaking those thought patterns that are holding us back from having a conversation, and it can inform the conversation we have when we do actually speak to them.'

7. Precious things

The role of our belongings in belonging

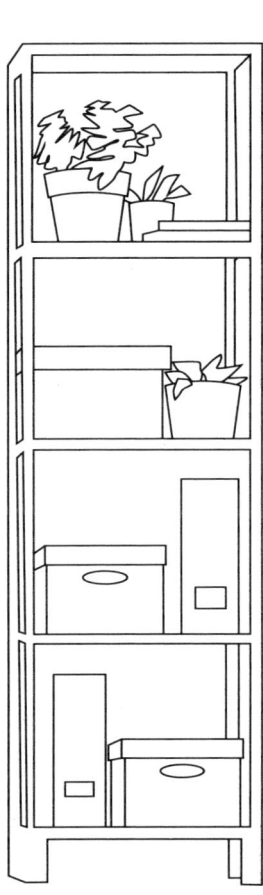

"Have nothing in your houses which
you do not know to be useful or believe
to be beautiful"
William Morris[1]

The IKEA bags are never far away. Those glossy, bright blue ones with thick, scratchy handles have become a symbol of upheaval for me. Having trusted these vast, heavy-duty bags to carry my belongings between eight different house shares now, I can feel the sting of the red indentations they leave on my hands just thinking about them.

When I think about where 'home' has been for me in the past 10 years, it isn't one room, house, or flat I think of. It's the collection of belongings I've unpacked in each space I've occupied. Without an attachment to one place, I instead think of these IKEA bags and the things I put inside them, which have the power to make anywhere feel more homely to me. Sturdy and durable, these bags have held my home-making kit. My own transportable version of home.

I'm in my 30s now, carrying one of these giant blue bags in each hand, and the stinging sensation is setting in as I walk towards the door of my eighth house share. Lamps and cushions are balanced precariously at the top, while my books and weighty picture frames sit down at the bottom.

This is the point when I'm returning to house sharing after living with a partner for two years. Despite that sabbatical, the muscle memory kicks in and, without a second thought, I'm going through the steps of setting up my room as I've always done. Clean the space before carrying the bags in, unpack, arrange my things corner by corner. It's now a fine art.

I unpack, holding each item in my hands before deciding where it should go, and reflect on the fact that, despite the different locations, housemates, room shapes, and walls in varying states of disrepair, this collection of stuff I've carried with me has been a thread of continuity through each space I've lived in. Our things can be what anchor us in places that would otherwise feel meaningless.

A personal anchor

According to psychologist, Christian Jarrett, our relationship with stuff and things starts at a young age – as early as two years old.[2] By the age of six,[3] we begin to value things more simply because they belong to us. I think back to my own childhood bedroom, and look at how my young nephews and nieces adorn their bedrooms with their belongings. It's clear to see how, during those childhood years, the room where you sleep becomes a treasure trove of precious things: stickers from school covering bed frames, certificates and posters covering the walls, collections of fossils and toys covering every available surface.

Psychologists talk about 'transitional objects' as the ones that children are most attached to as they gradually make the move away from their parents towards being independent.[4] We call them security blankets or toys because they offer a sense of safety and familiarity as we grow up and, eventually, move out from the family home.

Then, as we grow older, the things we value change, but our relationships with the objects we own strengthen. They are like physical memories, reminders of who we are, where we've come from, experiences we've had.

For most of us, it is these things and objects that make a home feel like *our* home. We find an empty shell of a place – flats, houses, bought, rented, or shared – and fill the shelves with our books, and adorn the walls with prints and art we like, and, suddenly, it feels more like our space. A blank slate we've put our stamp on.

When you're house sharing, your things are the *only* way you can put your stamp on a space. You can't paint, renovate, or change the space dramatically. The only way to make it feel less like a blank slate is to fill it with your stuff. I always feel that my attachment to the things I put in my room in a house share is heightened somehow. The term 'transitional objects' has taken on a new meaning for me. Now, they're not the things that helped me to feel safe as I gained independence from my mum, transitional objects are the things that bring me a sense of safety as I move from house share to house share. They are the things I connect with, invest in, and surround myself with, offering me security amid a lot of house moves. They allow me to shift from feeling 'stuck' in a house share to carving out my own independent version of home in a shared space.

Our belongings play a role in our emotional wellbeing and how settled and secure we feel. It's a relationship that Eugene Halton, a former professor of sociology at the University of Notre Dame in Indiana, USA, and co-author of *The Meaning of Things*, has researched in great detail. I ask him for his insights into how the stuff we own impacts the way we feel day to day. 'We really project and extend ourselves in things and derive a sense of self from the things we own as well', he says. 'Our objects are mirrors that tell us who we are and, at the same time, they can act as instruments and role models for how you want to be.'

Right now, this room in my eighth house share feels wholly unfamiliar. It doesn't hold any memories yet. Other rooms I've lived in started to feel like home because I'd found respite or solace there. I haven't made that connection to this one yet. This room doesn't offer me stability or any promise of permanence, and I don't feel connected to the housemate living here either. My things, though, offer me some continuity and connection. They are tangible objects that I recognise and can hold. Something that's familiar when everything around me is new.

I have called this room my own for a matter of hours, but just the presence of my belongings, and the memories that come with them, means I begin to see it as home. A study by Jane Kroger, Professor of Psychology at UiT, the Arctic University of Norway in Tromsø, and Dr Vivienne Adair, a developmental psychologist and lecturer at Auckland University, New Zealand, looks at the symbolic meaning of personal objects for people in later adulthood who have relocated.[5] They interviewed 20 adults in New Zealand, who were between the ages of 65 and 89 and had moved from their own homes to supervised housing for older people. Their objects became of paramount importance, reminding them of who they were and their history as their home environment changed. Jane and Vivienne concluded that 'objects served the function of providing a personal kind of anchor in times of change' and 'were concrete physical reminders of who the participant was, who he or she is now and how he or she is connected across time and place to present, past and future generations and eras'.

Unlike the flat where I lived with a partner and filled every cupboard and corner with my belongings, having less stuff to sort out this time does feel calming in a way I hadn't anticipated. I feel quite free knowing that, if tomorrow something arises and I have to move on, I can. I think about the trend for tiny living – people choosing to live in very small homes, wanting to live a simple, sustainable, and portable life. 'If you own a property or live with a partner, you're going to feel more restricted if or when you want to move on,' observes psychologist Professor Stephen Palmer, Founder Director of the Centre for Stress Management in London. 'Whereas a house share does present a freedom where you can make that decision yourself and escape the interpersonal pressures quite easily if it's too much to cope with.'

Having just a room's worth of belongings certainly streamlines my choices: I only wear what I've brought with me here, I only read the books that could fit in. And there is something calming and liberating about knowing that, if I had to move, I could throw my belongings into those IKEA bags and pick my life up quite easily.

What's mine is mine

As I unpack, I get pangs of nostalgia and flashbacks to the last time I moved. It was with Noah, my boyfriend at the time, into a one-bedroom flat where we lived just us as a couple. We'd had the whole flat to fill and, as we moved our stuff in, we had conversations about how we'd spruce it up – get fresh curtains for the bedroom, ask the landlord if we could paint the kitchen, get a big plant for the bathroom, hang pictures and create photo walls in the living room.

Here, though, the communal spaces are already filled with things that belong to the existing housemate and those who came before. The shelves are lined with books that don't belong to me, no room for mine. The cupboards are packed with kitchen gear. The only empty shell that's left for me to put my stamp on is the bedroom I'm renting. Even here, I have to work with the brilliant white walls that are scuffed in places and the slightly stained carpet. The bed and mattress have been in the room for years. But it is here, in the limited ways available to me, that I can arrange my things and make it feel like my place.

Eugene tells me about a study he conducted, asking people which room they felt the most at home in. 'The adults said the kitchen or living room, but for the teenagers and children, it was overwhelmingly the bedroom that was most important to them, where they felt most at home. And it was because they had freedom, away from their parents and in their own space. Like crustaceans, able to form a new skin under the shell of the home. The privacy was really important. And these are aspects, I think, that would reappear in a house sharing situation – where the privacy your room offers you becomes overwhelmingly important.'

House sharing feels infantilising at times. In the same way that children are free to decorate the walls of their bedrooms with things that feel meaningful to them, but not the communal spaces, us house sharers can do what we will with our rooms, but the communal spaces remain out of bounds. Despite being adults, the parameters set are frightfully similar to those we might have experienced in our childhoods.

I decide I'll store certain things in my room, to protect them. A childlike possessiveness kicks in because, in a space where we can control very little, the stuff we have and *can* control feels important.

When everything in your home is shared, the things you own that are just yours become disproportionately valuable. Everyone has their own thing in a house share that they want to protect from communal usage or, worse, someone else breaking it. For me, it's a collection of mugs I've picked up from vintage markets and little shops over the years. I protect those things here, in this house share, more than I ever did when I lived with my partner.

Over the years, I've noticed other housemates doing the same with their things. One woman I shared with kept her KitchenAid mixer in her room, only bringing it out when she wanted to bake. Another stored her pink Le Creuset casserole dish on top of the fridge, with strict instructions that we needed to ask before using it. It's interesting that the items people invest in signify adulthood – like the nice mixer and casserole dish. By protecting the usage of these things, it's as though we are protecting the small slice of adulthood that we have access to.

Interestingly, research has discovered a link between low self-esteem (how we value ourselves) and an increase in materialism. The researchers noticed how, when self-esteem was at its lowest, participants were more likely to use material possessions as part of a coping strategy to deal with insecurities.[6] 'As children mature into teens, we see possessions starting to act as a crutch for the self,' says psychologist Christian Jarrett, talking about the study in his article in *The Psychologist*, mentioned earlier in this chapter. I can see that there's a similar link between house sharers' self-esteem and materialism. A house share – a space defined by communal living and compromise – challenges how we value and perceive ourselves, so has an impact on our self-esteem. A house sharing set-up can undermine the autonomy that comes with adulthood and so we might find ourselves using material objects to steady ourselves. While others might feel in some way defined by their home or where they live as a space where they express themselves through their décor, house sharers only have their own belongings at their disposal to serve this purpose.

This link between self-esteem and material objects explains why, when someone breaks something of ours or uses it, it hits harder in the house sharing environment than it generally would if you were in your own home because, whether we realise it or not, it is so closely linked to how we see and perceive ourselves in the world. Alongside this, there's the related element of feeling in control. In a living environment where we often feel at the mercy of others, our possessions are some of the only things we *can* control, so if something happens to them, it can feel as though that control has been taken away, which can be incredibly destabilising. Our reactions to such events may sometimes seem irrational to others not in the same living situation as us, but make perfect sense to anyone who understands just how precious our possessions are in a shared space.

'It's helpful to look at the thinking behind anger and stress that arise when a housemate uses your things,' says Stephen. 'Often, we won't have shared our rules or demands with others, so they might not know they're breaking our rules by using our things. My approach to this in coaching would be to use realistic thinking. So your starting point might be, "My housemate shouldn't use my mug. I can't stand it when they do", but you can change that to, "It's preferable that my housemate doesn't use my mug, but if they do, I can stand it." It's a rational approach that means we can be more forgiving and acknowledge how our own rules and set beliefs are fuelling our frustrations.'

Protecting your space

Part of the process of claiming your space in a house share – alongside finding a place for your things – is creating somewhere that calms us and offers a place of recuperation. I ask Saskia Wheeler, a brand consultant specialising in neuroaesthetics (how what we see around us affects our brain, body, and behaviour) what we can do in a house share to create a space that feels more like home.

'For most of us, "being at home" means having space to breathe,' she says. 'That can be difficult to achieve when house sharing because, when we share a space with others, we can sometimes pick up on their stress and that makes it more challenging to create a space that maintains lower levels of stress in the body. If the only private space is your room, then make it one that's tranquil and peaceful. We tend to associate spaces with certain thought patterns. So, if you're escaping to your room because you don't have a great relationship with your housemates, then it might become a place you end up ruminating, and then those unhelpful thought processes fester. As much as you can, try to safeguard your room from those thought processes – going to meet a friend or for a walk to process them instead – so it doesn't become a place with negative associations.'

It's the kind of advice I've heard sleep specialists give to people who struggle to get to sleep – that you should leave your bedroom and only return when you feel ready for sleep. Otherwise, it becomes a place you associate with stress, which is not conducive to good sleep.

I also ask Saskia what we can do to protect our rooms in house shares and keep them as spaces that feel stress-free. 'If you find yourself constantly ruminating in your space, finding some way to practise gratitude is a really good way to reframe your thinking to create a more positive outlook. Our brains can't appreciate and feel fear at the same time. Keep a notepad somewhere and write a journal or a list of a few things you're grateful for that day. If you're able to make it a habit, it can help to offset that cycle of rumination your brain might otherwise slip into.'

There are some other things you can do to reset. Saskia says taking practical steps can be really powerful. 'We know that nature-inspired design can help to lower stress levels, so having plants, calm and serene lighting, such as low, tonal hues in the evening, and natural woods can help to create a space that feels more calming. Listening to positive music helps too. Studies have shown that when people listen to their favourite music, this increases levels of the pleasure-inducing hormone dopamine in the body.

'Try to introduce activities that increase levels of dopamine and serotonin in the body. Try to mitigate exposing yourself to blue light, which can lower levels of dopamine throughout the day. Read a book, write in your journal, do something creative that's cognitively rewarding. These are a few ways of helping to reset your space, but so much of it is about reinforcing positive thought patterns to try and drive up levels of these happy hormones. Things like worrying, ruminating, and socially isolating oneself can hardwire negative patterns of thought that can lead to overproduction of cortisol (stress hormone) and increased amygdala activity (fear and anxiety centre in the brain).'

House shares, by their very nature, challenge the traditional sense of home. They're temporary, not something we own, and not entirely private. If you're finding it challenging to cultivate a sense of belonging and create a space to recuperate, it's entirely understandable. But if we think of home as more of a process, of practising the art of making a home to create somewhere we associate with calm, and fill it with the meaning held in our belongings, this will help the space to become more meaningful to us. Doing this will free us from the idea that we are 'stuck' in a house share so, instead, we can believe we're cultivating a 'home for now', as we are surrounded by things that both anchor us and signify a hopeful future – whether that is in a house share or otherwise.

Thing-stories

In his book, Eugene talks about the role that 'thing-stories' play in our lives: 'In the beginning, there is creation. In the end, there is property. In the middle, there are thing-stories: thing-stories that throw light on the often fantastic ways in which we people our environments with objects, especially the domestic environment.'[8]

Thing-stories are the stories of the experiences, memories, relationships, habits, hobbies, studies and everything else attached to the physical items we own. Our things, in turn, tell a story of the things we find meaningful in the world. They show the places we've visited, with the people we value, and the art, films, and books that resonate with us.

Beth Jones is 29, has been house sharing since she was 23, and has lived in five house shares so far. 'I've always lived in house shares, so I don't have that much stuff because I can't spread out over the whole house like you might if you have a whole place. When I first moved into a house share, I remember my friends gifting me mugs with my name on and a wine glass with my name on as house-warming gifts. I was really protective over them. I didn't want anyone else to use them and, if they did, I'd be like, "Oh, my God. You're using my wine glass with my name on or my teacup that Emma got me!" We'd have our own cutlery, cups, cupboard, food – everything was kept separate. But then I'd find it really cute when a housemate said, "My mum got me this mug, but you can use it" – it felt like a real honour because I think, in a house share, you know how important these things are.'

Our objects, then, can become tools that we can use in various ways to shape our identities. As Eugene says, 'Our belongings are also instruments and role models for how you want to live and can help you realise or achieve certain goals.' Therefore, as we saw earlier in this chapter, we might protect our items, reinforcing that we have ownership of them, to satisfy an emotional need to exert at least some level of control in our living situation. And if we then choose to share those belongings with someone, it suggests that we no longer feel out of control around that person. We can afford to relax and let them cross our boundaries in these small ways, building connection.

I'm reminded of when I was living in the Balham house share with Phoebe, Jess, and Sophie. We've been making do with a table and four chairs that, every few weeks, we have to duct tape back together. You're lucky if you pick one of the two chairs that are sturdy enough to sit on, but one of the others falls apart as soon as you put weight on it and the remaining one is only fine if you keep your weight evenly spread between its four legs – shuffle and it'll collapse. It is a quite nice faux pine set, cheap and inoffensive, that was left by one of the previous house sharers who had lived in the flat I don't know how many years ago. We never really sit at the table, it's so unsteady. Instead, we eat on the sofas with our plates on our laps, to save the kerfuffle of trying to find the safe chair to perch on.

I don't know what switched for me at this point. Perhaps it is because this is the first house share where I feel like I have any say in what happens in the communal space. Or perhaps it's that, now I've been house sharing for seven years, and can't see a path out of it, I might as well make the best of it. Or perhaps it's that I feel a little bit sick about how many cheap IKEA flat-packs I've built and then later taken to a charity shop. Whatever it is, I decide that I should invest in furniture that I'll want to keep.

So I trawl Facebook Marketplace, looking for pre-loved things that I'd keep, wherever I go next. Choosing things that I could see in my future went some way to satisfying this yearning I had to make a home, something that, so far, had been repressed while I'd been living in house shares, where everything felt transient and I was unable to make my mark.

I buy a set of drawers for my room. And then, I find a pre-loved pine table for £50 that's currently sitting in someone's family home. It looks very much like the one I sat around at mealtimes as a child, with turned wooden legs that taper a little at the bottom. It's cheaper than anything I can find on IKEA's website and a few others I try, so I offer the £50 and organise for a courier van to pick it up.

I'm waiting for the driver to pull up outside the house. The departing table's been picked up, so there's a space ready and waiting for the new one. I'm running down the stairs to meet the driver when it dawns on me that the entrance door to our flat upstairs is very narrow. I walk over to say 'Hi' to the driver, who, thanks to the app, I know is called Dave.

'It was a nightmare getting this table out of the last place,' he says. 'I hope you've got a wide corridor.'

He's kindly offering to help me up to the flat with the table. I insist that I can take it from here – my housemates will give me a hand when they're home from work – but he wants to help. 'Come on, let's go,' he says.

I'm shuffling backwards towards the front door and then we hit a problem: it won't fit through. 'Have you got a screwdriver?' he says.

'Yes! I'll go and get it.'

So here we are, standing on the path that leads to the front door, in the dark, with fine, drizzly rain coming down. I shine the light from my phone torch on the corners of the table while Dave unscrews the legs.

One of my housemates, Phoebe, gets home from work and isn't sure what to make of it. She laughs and offers to take one of the detached legs upstairs. She comes back for the others.

Dave and I upend the tabletop and we cautiously carry it up the stairs to our flat, which is on the second floor. Finally, albeit in pieces, the table is in situ. Phoebe and I set about reconstructing it, Dave holding it in place.

Three hours after the delivery slot I'd booked, Dave, Phoebe, and I are sitting round the table I paid £50 for with cups of tea.

That table and its thing-story gave us a place to dine like the young adults we were, to host dinners, to play board games, to display a vase of flowers. For Sophie to do her paint-by-numbers kits and for us to work at on the occasional day we worked from home.

I took two days of annual leave to upcycle that table, sanding off the varnish with a sanding mouse my brother-in-law lent me and showed me how to use. I bought a couple of tester pots of lovely green paint and turned the legs green. It was the first piece of upcycling I'd ever done and I loved it. I knew all along that wherever I moved next, I'd take that table.

When I moved from that flat, I did take the table with me and, in the same way that transitional objects offer children stability, it saw me through a great deal of change and allowed me to hold on to the fact that, wherever I lived, I'd have a table to sit at and eat my meal like a grown-up. Last year, I sold it on the same website where I'd bought it from. I didn't need it in my eighth house share because my housemate already had a steadfast dining table with matching chairs in situ – as good a sign as any that I'm getting better at finding house shares with good housemates.

There are two different types of materialism that Eugene talks about. He says, 'I came up with a distinction between what I call instrumental materialism versus terminal materialism. Instrumental materialism is this idea that an object can serve as a means to realise a goal. They are materials with meaning. Terminal materialism is where the object is taken as an end in itself, more of an abstract prop. Where the ownership of that object is the end goal, it's the everyday sense of materialism rather than materials that have meaning. Materialism in this sense is really a mentalism, a domination by ideas rather than the things per se. So perhaps we need to become more materialistic. More aware in the sense of actually connecting to the material qualities of the things we surround ourselves with and the meanings they hold.'

Chapter reflections

How can you carve out your own independent version of home?
Are there bits of furniture, or prints, or pictures that you can envisage keeping with you when you move on? How can you create that feeling of home in ways that are transportable?

Can you think of ways you could keep your room as a recuperating space?
If you find yourself spending a lot of time in there with negative thoughts, are there ways you can process these differently and keep your room as a place to rest and recuperate?

How have you adapted to live in the space? How have you adapted the space for how you live?
Having a relationship with your room is part of connecting with it. Are there changes you've made to how you live to suit the space? Perhaps you've created a boundary between private and shared belongings. Or moved your plants to where they will get the right levels of light. And what have you done to change the space to suit you? Perhaps you've hung some different curtains or created a colour scheme you like with your furnishings. Strike a balance between adapting to the space and adapting it to you.

In what ways have you practised the art of making a home?
Perhaps you've displayed your things on a shelf or you've bought a rug to brighten the room. In what ways have you connected with the space to make it feel more like yours?

How do your own thing-stories shape your space?

Identify some of the objects around you that you feel anchor you. What are their thing-stories? What is it about them that makes you feel at home?

8. Dating by committee

Boundaries and benefits
of dating in a house share

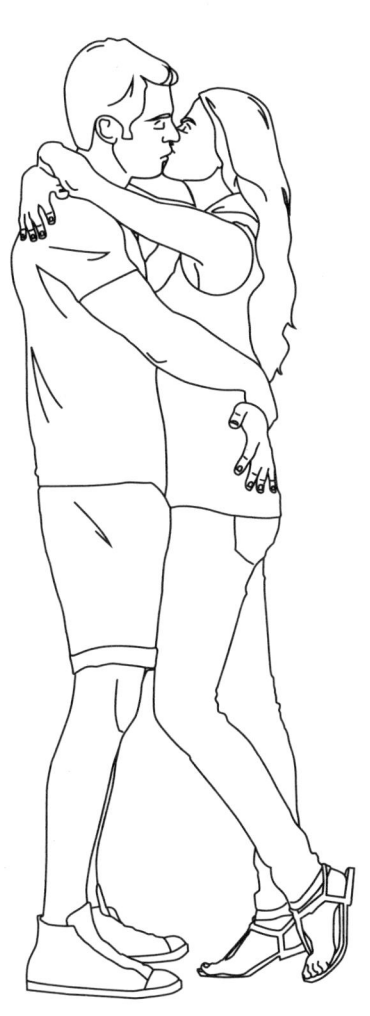

"Everyone has three lives: a public life,
a private life, and a secret life"
Gabriel García Márquez[1]

New words like 'ghosting', 'love bombing', 'situationships', and 'breadcrumbing' started appearing in conversations with my friends when I was in my 20s. Before they were coined, there were simply no words that accurately described the web of confusion that is modern dating. And then, after learning about them, I'd watch each new word play out in my house shares right in front of my eyes. If breadcrumbing or love bombing wasn't happening to me personally, it was happening to one of my housemates, and I'd know every detail, so it was as though it was happening to me. When you live in a house share, dating is not a private affair.

This living situation provides an ideal springboard and support system for dating as being single is almost a prerequisite for house sharing. When you're coupled up in a long-term relationship, it's likely your house sharing days are almost over. So, I've lived alongside other single people in all my house shares. If you have, too, then you'll know how it feels to be navigating the dating scene together.

For me, there are benefits. Having a constellation of women around you means that, on the occasions when dates rearrange, cancel, flake, disappoint, or full-on ghost, someone's usually around to pick you up and take your mind off it. Or to help you come up with comforting but completely unrealistic explanations for the ghosting. And housemates can be your best cheerleaders – by your side when things are going well, present when you want to air something you're not sure about, and offering gentle encouragement when you need it. They are a network of people in your home who know only too well the excitement and challenges that dating presents. Advice on tap and a safety net for when things go wrong. This is, on paper, the ideal place to launch from into a budding romantic relationship.

But, dating in a house share also robs you of the privacy you want and need while you're getting to know another human intimately. You have to field opinions you haven't asked for. Awkward moments you never want anyone to know about are broadcast live in your house share for all housemates to witness. And you probably know as well as I do that it's virtually impossible to keep your sex life private when your rooms are separated by a stud wall.

If modern dating generally is a maze, then dating in a house share is a labyrinth of potential issues that we have to navigate as sensitively as possible.

Date nights in house shares

I'm thinking back to my Balham house share again. Watching a film with Phoebe, Jess, and Sophie, I match with Finn on Bumble – the Irish yoga teacher you might remember me mentioning in Chapter 1. He's three years older than me and, conveniently, works at the yoga studio down the road from our flat. After my initial 'Hey', he's been chatty and responsive. Our messages are short and frequent – a pace we're both excited and dedicated enough to keep up.

When Phoebe goes to top our wine up, I pass my phone to Sophie to show her my latest match. She flicks through the profile with ease, knowing her way around the app from her own dating forays. She looks closely at his three pictures. There's one of him doing a headstand and another of him on a sofa with his mate, smiling. On seeing the one of him at the finishing line of a running race, lifting his little niece up, with the caption 'Not my kid', she does a little eyeroll and smiles.

'Yeah he looks nice. Seems sporty, family orientated... What's the chat like?'

'He seems pretty funny, yeah.'

I smile and take my phone back. It matters to me that my housemates agree he looks like a good guy. I arrange to meet him that Friday after work. Finn messages me over the app as I'm walking over to the pub down one of the side streets opposite my office.

'I'm wearing a hat and yellow Converse x'

Walking over, I can see his hat and yellow Converse. He's sitting on a bench outside. I take a breath and smile, preparing myself for a forced conversation, but really hoping it'll be a good, flowing one.

'Hey,' I say and wait for him to look up and confirm I've got the right person.

'Hiya,' he says. He's just the right amount of smiley. Smooth, casual but genuine.

It's crowded, so we perch on the same side of the bench, turning towards each other to chat. I'm getting a waft of his woody aftershave every time he leans forward to say something. I'm relieved that the conversation is coming easily, because it's distracting me from how close and intimate it feels. We're talking non-stop, only breaking to order another round of pints.

When he calls a few days later, as promised, I conceal how excited I am to hear from him. I like that we're talking over the phone rather than texting. I like the sound of his voice and the conversation. It makes me more sure of him, and so we meet again. And again. And before long, we've fallen into a pattern of seeing each other mid-week and then once at the weekend. He calls me most days in between the yoga classes he's teaching. He's open with his emotions and we're having a lot of fun going to sound baths and random gigs around London together.

It's two months or so into dating and I've invited him over for dinner. Tonight's the first time I'm cooking a curry from scratch for us, and there are so many spices and fresh ingredients to chop that I keep getting it wrong. I'm flustered because the recipe's a bit complicated and, despite putting feelers out earlier in the week and deciding that no one would be in tonight, two out of my three housemates are also in the kitchen cooking. Finn and I will have to eat in my room if we want some privacy.

So, I set up the tiny fold-up outdoor table and chairs I have in my room. With a bit of mood lighting and a candle, it's quite romantic. But, still, not quite the first dinner date at mine I'd hoped for. Finn arrives when, thankfully, I'm less flustered, but then we have to do three trips up the stairs with the wine, water, and plates of food. Still, it's cosy, we chat more, and I forget all about accidentally adding six garlic cloves instead of three. He stays over that night and when I wake up in the morning – the smell of curry still lingering in the air – I feel a bit on edge about whether Sophie heard us having sex. I'd been lost in the moment after Finn and I had drunk a lot of wine, so my memory's hazy, but I know how thin the wall is between my room and hers because I've heard her sex noises multiple times.

Finn leaves to teach his first yoga class of the weekend. I let him out the front door and, on the way back to my room – bleary-eyed, with last night's mascara crumbling off my lashes, I bump into Phoebe in the kitchen.

PHOEBE: 'Finn seems really nice, Al.'

ME: 'Yeah, he does, doesn't he?'

PHOEBE: 'So, do you know where it's going? Have you had that chat?'

ME: 'Ooh no. Not yet. Just seeing how it goes, I guess.'

PHOEBE: 'Yeah, it's been a while though, right? Just make sure he's not taking you for a ride.'

Then Phoebe leaves to meet her friend for a coffee.

I haven't really thought about possibly being hurt yet. We're still getting to know each other and I'm trying very hard, which anyone in the throes of dating knows isn't easy, not to project too far into the future. I'm wanting to keep things realistic, but now I'm worrying that Phoebe can see something I can't.

There's a term psychologists use to describe the first stage of a romantic relationship – usually the first six months. It's 'symbiosis'[2] and it describes what happens in the period of time when two individuals come together to explore how compatible they are before deciding to merge into a 'we'. It's the stage between a couple meeting and becoming exclusive. The stage when it might seem that they're prioritising each other over other things in their lives as they build a foundation that will drive their relationship forward. It's also the stage when spending time together alone is important.

In a house share, not only is creating that physical time and space a challenge but so, too, is creating the mental space to decide what's right for you while also considering your housemates' needs and opinions. Finn and I were only two months into dating and already I felt that our relationship was being unavoidably shaped by my house share.

Five's a crowd

The next time I saw Finn after Phoebe had asked about our future as a couple, I was on edge. I started reading too much into what it was we were doing, what he wanted, and whether we were heading towards a committed relationship or if he was dating other people at the same time. Phoebe's questioning had – for the right or wrong reasons – burst the bubble I'd been living in for the past couple of months.

In a house share where you, willingly or not, share details about your dating life, you're engaging in something that therapists term 'triangulation'. You're drawing someone else into the dynamic you have as a couple, and that can bring both positives and negatives. On the one hand, you get a second opinion and support, and someone holds you accountable to your own goals and personality. It can be very comforting to have that in the early stages of dating, when a relationship can feel fragile as you're working out what you want from it.

On the other hand, the downside is that the advice your housemate gives you is going to be bound up with their own individual experiences, so it isn't always good, reliable advice that will be relevant to you. It can also cause a breakdown in communication between the person you're dating and you. Whether you realise it or not, you can end up breaking the trust between you by holding on to the opinions of people outside the relationship. Other peoples' anxieties can end up muddying your thoughts.

In my situation with Finn, I felt like I was carrying my housemate's anxieties as well as my own. I couldn't really give Finn a reason for my anxiety, other than the fact that it was something my housemate had said. In the end, he ended things after nine months, not wanting to start a relationship when he knew he wanted to move back to Ireland. Perhaps I would have found that out earlier if I'd listened to Phoebe, but I needed the space to see where the relationship was going for myself.

There's a fine balance to be achieved between caring about what your housemates think and not falling victim to their judgements. I ask psychotherapist, author, and podcaster Emma Reed Turrell for advice on how to handle the friend–date dichotomy. 'When you hear an opinion from a housemate,' she says, 'observe it and be separate from it and still care, but don't get enmeshed in it. If they pass a judgement on your dating situation, can you be curious about it? Have a healthy amount of emotional detachment from their opinions. Then ask yourself, "Is there a seed of truth?" And is there anything you can learn from your emotional response to their opinion?'

Sophia Hilton, 32, works in marketing and has lived in four house shares – two in Cambridge and two in London – where she's navigated her own romantic relationships alongside those of her housemates. 'The thing is, as a housemate, you see behind closed doors – all the facets of a relationship you wouldn't normally see. I've known more about my housemates' relationships than I've ever known about my close friends who are in long-term relationships. Because, living with them, I know the good, the bad, and the ugly. You see how often they're seeing each other, you hear laughter through the wall, or you hear shouting through the wall, or you hear bickering. All of it. And you wouldn't invite that level of exposure into your relationship normally or even talk about it in that level of detail with your friends.

'It does then somehow give the housemate on the outside of the relationship the justification for asking questions or giving their opinion quite strongly because they feel like they're in it. Times I've been going into something new, or even times I've gone through break-ups, and I've not been quite sure where I'm at with it. I don't want opinions; I've wanted the space to figure it out for myself. Housemates can always put the puzzle together without you actually having to say anything. It's hard because you do want to keep a level of privacy for your relationship, like you do from your friends and your family.'

In the first house share Sophia lived in, during her early 20s, she moved in when she was already in an established relationship. They broke up and got back together while she was there and she felt the need to justify her decisions to her housemates. 'They'd witnessed the break-up and, when you break up with somebody, you naturally say all of the bad bits. And they'd been there for me. But then, when we got back together, I felt like I had to work hard at reintroducing my boyfriend to them. I was trying to convince my housemates that it was the right thing and he was a good person. I had to do it carefully, but also lay it on quite thick for a long time. I felt I had to explain my decisions and overemphasise anything good he did or that we did together because I wanted my housemates to be OK with him being there again, despite all I'd said about him when we broke up. It was kind of exhausting. I panicked about him changing the dynamic in the house and I worried about losing my core group of friends in the house share in case my relationship didn't work out. My people-pleasing tendencies got the better of me, as I think they do for a lot of women my age in house shares. And, actually, looking back, me prioritising the house share probably did affect my relationship a little.'

Psychotherapist Emma works with people-pleasers every day in her clinical practice, so I ask her to share her insights. 'I think a lot of young women feel held back by people-pleasing tendencies,' she observes, 'and I can see how, in a house share scenario where you're dating, too, it can complicate your experience.

'Before you begin dating, get really clear on where your house share relationships sit. One of the things I talk about as part of my anti-people-pleasing manifesto is your rings of relationships. Get clear on who is in the centre of that circle of relationships: they're those really close relationships that can sometimes seem fragile because they mean so much to you. You don't want to go blazing in there with your size eights on, destroying that relationship with your new-found kind of "please yourself" mentality. Outside of that, there might be extended friendships, outside of that there might be colleagues, outside of that there might be somebody in the supermarket. Each layer less significant. You can practise pleasing yourself in the outer layers. So, saying to the person in the supermarket, "Actually, I don't know if you noticed, but I was ahead of you in the queue." That's where you get to practise pleasing yourself. And then you can come in a layer and get more evidence that you can please yourself and not destroy relationships. Then you work your way in until you're actually able to say to your mother – at the centre of your rings – "We see things differently. And that's OK." What your housemates think about your dating habits or potential new partner is probably going to be less important to you than what your friend of 20 years thinks. And perhaps it's OK that you see things differently.

'Short term, it may cause tension in your home and mean you need to navigate the awkwardness and discomfort that comes with that but, longer term, it's likely your housemates' opinion of your date isn't going to be something keeping you up at night. It might allow you to take a risk, to navigate some of your identity development inside a relationship that's less significant to you, where the consequences of you taking the risk to please yourself aren't so dire.'

Chances are, everyone will have different dating goals and habits. Over the years, I've lived with housemates looking for a serious relationship, people casually dating multiple people, those who just wanted the odd fling now and then, some with experimental sex lives who loved talking about them, and people who hated talking about their dating lives – and other people's. In a house share where sexual habits, preferences, and relationship goals are wildly different, it can be hard to find a balance that works for everyone – particularly when it comes to overnight stays.

Let's talk about sex

In my interviews with the people for this book, sex and dating stories usually began with a grimace. One woman described turning on the light on the landing to go to the toilet in the middle of the night and bumping into her housemate's one-night stand. Naked. Another described having her housemate's boyfriend try to get in bed with her at 2am because he'd got the wrong bedroom. Then there were multiple stories of people being kept up all night by the banging of a bed or scratching of a headboard. Then there were the vivid descriptions of sex sounds coming from housemates' bedrooms, ranging from 'whimpering dog' to 'whale sounds' to grunts. Then there were the ones of awkwardness. Seeing your housemate and the guy she'd just started dating leaving the bathroom after having a shower together, knowing that they'd probably done more than lather shower gel on each other. Getting home to find your housemate and her new partner having sex on the kitchen table. Sitting on a work conference call trying to present while hearing your housemate climax at 11am on a Tuesday.

'I find intimacy really awkward in a house share,' says Sophia. 'I absolutely hate the thought of anybody hearing anything. There was a bit of an issue in one house share where, basically, there was a space between the floorboards between our rooms, so me and my housemate Julia could hear our other housemate Becky having sex. She was casually dating at that point, so it was once a week at least. It was awkward, but it didn't bother me because I was like, "What can she do?" There's nothing she can do. But it used to really grate on Julia, and she'd not talk to Becky the next day because it was too loud and she was annoyed about it but wouldn't say anything. And, actually, Julia had a boyfriend and I remember her saying that she never slept with him in the house share because she was worried about people hearing her. I think she was saying it because she thought we should all do the same. But what can you do when that's your home?'

Boiling it down to the impact it's having on you is a good way to approach conversations about disruptive sex. So, if you're feeling unsafe because your housemate is bringing a lot of unknown people into the space, explain that you feel unsafe about strangers coming into the house. If the noise is affecting you, discuss the noise. If it's that you walked on to the landing to find their date naked, say that nudity in the communal spaces makes you feel uncomfortable. By thinking of how it's affecting you and opening a general conversation about that, rather than their sexual habits, you're preserving some privacy and not passing judgement.

'Maybe it is appropriate to dial down sexual activity in a house full of adults who also want to sleep and go to work,' says Emma. 'As adults living alongside one another, I don't think you can judge the noise differently because it's sex. But you do get to call it out because it's noise. Noise is noise. You probably would feel fine bringing up the fact that someone plays loud music at all hours or hoovers at 5am on a Sunday. So it stands to reason that if the grunting or the bed shaking or the banging headboard is disruptive, you can address it as a noise issue.'

A safety net

A good house share is the place to be when you're a single person. The years I was single, house shares I lived in meant that I was surrounded by people to socialise and explore London with. The things that coupled-up friends did with their partners, I did with my housemates: morning run and coffee at the weekend, day trips, Sunday roasts. When the balance tipped for me and I started actively looking to meet a partner, being in house shares alongside other people doing the same offered a unique source of support and camaraderie from people who truly understood. With meaningful connections in my day-to-day life, it meant I could approach dating from a place of abundance and make good dating decisions.

During my 20s especially, I struggled to anchor myself after dating scenarios that left me feeling emotionally bruised. Having housemates in my life was a blessing. I never felt alone and, actually, just their physical presence as I made my way on my dating journey meant it felt like I always had people on my side.

'I suppose it's us recreating family where family doesn't exist,' says Emma. 'We've outgrown that family model of the past and have created a kind of peer group of our own. I have a client who has absolutely navigated dating with the support of the community of her house. She would say it got her out of a relationship that was toxic, it helped her rebuild her self-esteem, she had a group of people to come home to and talk to about how it'd gone. We often talk about the smoke and mirrors of the dating world, and we need real living, breathing humans to help us reality test what's going on sometimes. To be able to actually say, "Are you sure that's a real concern or is that your stuff?" Having that support means dating isn't this pressure cooker of messaging on apps. Instead, we have this way of testing that I think we need when we're figuring out our identity and dating and not always feeling 100 per cent secure in ourselves.'

Modern dating is brutal. Even as someone who thinks that they have at least some self-confidence, is a good judge of character, and is self-aware, I have fallen into every possible trap: I've misread signs, got tangled up with non-committal types I thought were serious, been swept off my feet by impressive people who were not particularly kind, pined over people who could barely make time to text me back, been too full on too early, and kept it so cool that I froze people out.

Dating is a treacherous road of self-discovery. If you care about people and you're emotionally available and vulnerable – all the things you need to be to meet someone and fall in love – then it has the ability to rock you to your very core.

'There's an accountability to dating that I quite like in the house share scenario,' says Emma. 'People see your behaviour, I suppose, like it would be in a family, but not something you necessarily want your mum to know. These people just see your comings and goings, and they see how you are when you come home, they see how you are over a cup of tea the next morning, and they can give you those little checking ins, which is what I think the family role would be. But we wouldn't want it from our actual family.'

During those years, as coupled-up friends started getting more serious and settling down into houses they'd bought and discussing having children, I felt less and less able to share my dating life with them. And so my housemates meant I had people I could talk about that stage with.

Sophia felt the same way as me. 'In a house share where others are dating, it just becomes part of your everyday. Going on a date is just part of your week, like going to the cinema. If I saw a friend for dinner and I was like, "Oh, I'm going on a date tomorrow," it'd be way bigger than me just saying to the house, "I'm going to the pub for a date tonight." My housemates put way less pressure on it. And if they're on the dating scene, too, they just get it. I might come home and say, "It just wasn't quite right," and we might chat about it at dinner for five minutes. Whereas if I went out for dinner with a friend, it'd sometimes be a half hour's conversation, which is more weight than I wanted to give it that early on.'

Having ended a long-term relationship, Sophia moved from Cambridge to London. 'Going back into a house share after a break-up was the best thing. I didn't feel alone and I had this safety blanket of a house share again. When I started dating again, if I had a bad date or things didn't go how I wanted, nine times out of 10 there was someone in the house to chat to and laugh about it. I immediately felt less rubbish. It stops you spiralling into feeling a bit lonely, downtrodden, or pessimistic. On the flip side, if it was a good date, it's nice to go home and tell somebody. I struggled a little bit with sharing dating stories with friends in very happy long-term relationships because sometimes their enquiring can come across as patronising, and sometimes you don't want to open up about your dating so soon with your friends. So, it's nice to go home and have somebody who just gets it, who you can debrief with.'

Shifting priorities

A time comes in any new relationship when a 'we' is more established. For me, when I've been living in a house share, that moment has tended to look like all my housemates knowing my boyfriend at kitchen chat level, his toothbrush being left at mine, us sharing our time between my place and his. It's meant that, for two or three nights a week, I've been either at his or he's been at mine. That unavoidably shifts the dynamic in the house share. No longer are you embedded in house share life, when you sit and eat together, watch films on a Friday night, and are readily available for spontaneous house share plans. Things have to be more carefully planned now that priorities are shifting.

It's a transitional period and it left me continually wondering whether I was making the right choices. It's a balancing act – trying to invest enough in your relationship to give it room to flourish, while also nurturing your housemate relationships in case it doesn't.

I return in my mind to my third year living in Balham with Phoebe, Sophie, and Jess. Things are approaching some level of normal after the pandemic, though we're still working from home. I've been dating Noah for three months now. He's an engineer, texts only once a day, but is consistent. After a little back and forth over the app we matched on, we moved to WhatsApp, then started going on long walks around London together when Covid lockdowns meant we couldn't go into each other's houses. He lived just the other side of Wandsworth

Common, so we would meet most days for a stroll and a coffee or a wine outside. Then restrictions were lifted and we'd stay at mine or his most nights.

I come back from his house one morning to set up for my day working from home. I walk into the lounge to find that my other housemates have set up their work laptops on the table but aren't there. They've gone to get coffee together. I stand there looking at their stuff. I'm annoyed I hadn't made it back in time to join them for the coffee run and think, 'Have they forgotten I'll need a space?' I go upstairs and set myself up in my room. When I hear them get back, chatting away about something they'd watched on TV last night, I go downstairs to say 'Hi'. But I can feel this icy energy.

Every time I return after staying at Noah's, I get the same feeling – that I'm missing out on something. There's some arrangement or a reference I don't get and have to ask for it to be explained. After a few weeks, I reach a point where I feel like I can't be an active member of the house share while also in a relationship. It feels impossible to hold the house share in the same space that I did before I met Noah. I'm struggling to find my place in my own home.

I ask Emma what's going on here. 'In a romantic relationship, we know about a term called "trauma bonding" – a deep connection that's formed when we face a distressing situation together. I suppose there could be some kind of intimacy bond that's created here in a house share between single women who are living alongside one another day in, day out. And then when someone gets into a romantic relationship, there comes a fear of loss.' When you're about to lose the house share as you know it and the housemate relationships might be about to change for good, it can feel threatening and you might start seeing that person differently, treading a bit carefully as you prepare for the change. 'Understanding and unpacking fear of loss as a potential blind spot can be really liberating. Underneath it all, what are you afraid of losing?' says Emma.

For me, I was afraid of losing that safety net of the house share and, potentially, that period of my life ending. Looking back, I needed to acknowledge that the choices I was making meant I was changing, my day-to-day life was changing, and therefore my relationships in the house were changing – and it was OK that things were changing.

'It doesn't sound very romantic or very friendly, but I think it boils down to contracting,' says Emma. 'There are some relationships in my life where I call myself a friendship freelancer. So, just like when you take a job and sign a freelance contract, the friendship works for a period of time and under certain conditions – so you might both be doing the same yoga course, for example. After that, when the contract ends, I don't hold those people to who they previously were, and I don't want to be held to that either. The nature of the freelance arrangement is that there's no shade if it stops working, but you can renegotiate for as long as it is. So the house share is a space where you're welcome as you are at that time and, in six months' time, you also want to be welcomed as you are. You might not be the same person or bring the same things to the table as you did in the first six months, so it's time to end that contract and begin a new one, with different terms and conditions. It's time to renegotiate the contract.

'It's important to be accountable and responsible too. So, yes, if your plans are changing or your life is changing and you've got into a relationship and it's going to have an impact on your housemate, be accountable for that and say, "I'm really sorry because I think this is having an impact on you, but I want to make this choice and I also want to acknowledge that that's having an impact on you. I recognise that and I see that."'

Sophia explains that she felt guilty getting into a relationship when one of her housemates was single because they used to spend a lot of time together. Now, there's a shift in how much time and energy she can give to the house share. 'Our relationship was one based on things we would do because we'd both be in on a Friday night and be like, "What are you doing tomorrow? Let's go for a coffee" kind of thing. We went on holidays and stuff, but it was very much chatting about it while we were working from home together. We both said we wanted to go to Amsterdam or Greece and then we just booked it. It was never intentional, just spontaneous. And now I'm in a relationship and that's changed. I don't have the same amount of free time.

'I feel a guilt. I don't want my housemate to have the worst year of her life living in a house as the only single person. I remember turning 30 and being single and all my friends were in long-term relationships and everyone was getting married. It was just so much and it felt like a massive milestone, so I felt very sad about it. I'm very conscious that she might be in the same headspace, so I don't want her to feel uncomfortable or sad in her own home. So I have started spending more and more time at my boyfriend's, to give her space to have her mates over and to date. I don't know if it makes it better or worse. Since I've started spending more time with my boyfriend, I've reached out to see if she wants to do a coffee or a brunch, but she just doesn't reply to me. And when I do go back to the flat, I get one-word answers from her. It's really hard not to feel pushed out.'

Shedding some light on what's going on here, Emma suggests how we might deal with any guilt that arises during this sort of transition. 'Get really clear on what your responsibility is and what it isn't.' What's your duty of care in this house share? It's important to recognise that it's not your responsibility to make your housemates feel comfortable. And that they are responsible for their response to things. It's about accountability. You follow your moral compass and be really clear on what that is. A genuine kind of evaluation of what you think is appropriate, not just one that works for you on that given day. Then decide what feels appropriate to you. Acting according to your moral compass is your 50 per cent. Then let the other person take their 50 per cent of responsibility to feed back.

'If you feel like you're making assumptions about what's going on for them, check it out. Say, "I was picking up on an atmosphere last night. Am I imagining that or am I on the right lines?" Showing our workings for a conclusion we've reached can help us do a bit of the bridge building for them and encourage them to feed back, to give us their 50 per cent. This is an adult relationship, not parent–child. The responsibility is 50:50.'

Dating someone who lives in a house share

When you're dating someone and their living environment is shared, too, it adds another layer to that initial phase of a relationship when you're getting to know each other. With men I've dated, when I've visited their house shares for the first time, I've always tried to make sure their housemates knew I was coming or, on first meeting, that the person I was dating and whose house share it was made proper introductions. It's something I also try to do for anyone new I'm dating when they visit my house share, as it alleviates some of the initial awkwardness.

Friends of mine describe feeling reluctant to ask a new date to have a conversation with their housemates to let them know they're coming over, not wanting to come across as 'too serious too early on'. But I think for them to introduce themselves to your housemates as someone you're dating is respectful, as doing this means that you or they don't then cause problems by simply being there. You're not asking them to put a definite label on things, but it can sometimes feel like a mini milestone as you're being invited or you're inviting them into another layer of your life.

Dan Smith, 30, lives in London and works in advertising. He describes how much pressure he felt when he met potential partners' housemates. 'It almost feels comparable to meeting your partner's family for the first time. It does feel like quite a big step. And it's quite a daunting thing. Because, often, at that stage, you don't know the relationship that they have and how much they talk to one another about things. You feel like you have to win *them* round as much as the person you're dating. And especially if you're looking to possibly spend more time in that flat, you don't want there to be rifts because you might be there more often. You want to make it as nice an experience as you can for the housemates.

'And when it comes to sex and getting intimate, the fact that the housemates are home is always at the forefront of my mind. It's such a private experience that you want it to be just you two. I remember, on certain occasions, for the first time, we wanted to make sure it was just us in the flat, so it could be private and we didn't have to worry about being quiet. That added layer of worrying can kind of ruin the whole atmosphere and the mood. It doesn't feel as relaxed or romantic.

'If I ever had to go to the bathroom, I'd be in my boxers and would listen out, then run as fast as I could to the bathroom, and I would just pray that they wouldn't come out at exactly the same time. Then there was this one time when I stayed over at a woman's house and, the evening I'd gone over, all the housemates were out, so I didn't meet them. But then, in the morning, they'd all come home. So I woke up and went down to the kitchen to get some water, not realising they were in, then met them for the first time on my own. I had to introduce myself to her housemates, like, "Hello, I'm Dan and I'm here with you know such and such. Good to meet you." It was so awkward. That's a big fear of mine now. If I'm dating someone who lives in a house share, I try to make sure I'm introduced to the housemates properly fairly early on, otherwise those encounters are so awkward.'

The truth is, even if your partner isn't particularly friendly with their housemates, you want to feel comfortable and relaxed in the space. But that's only really possible if you're properly introduced to those living there.

'It's always going to feel a little awkward to meet your new partner or date's housemates, so maybe the first step to navigating any awkwardness is to acknowledge it,' says Emma. 'You might choose to meet the housemates for a drink on neutral ground first, so that you're not stuck making polite conversation in the kitchen the morning after the night before. Or you might choose to chat to your date about how you've felt in the past when you've been introduced to your own housemates' love interests, then suggest that your date has a conversation to prepare their housemates for the fact that you will be around more often.'

When I first met Noah, we spent a lot of time in his house share as his three housemates didn't use the communal space. This meant that it was often free for us to cook in and watch films. But when one of the housemates was around, I'd feel hyper-aware that I was in their space and want to make sure that I wasn't imposing in any way. Even after a few months, I felt the same, so I'd try to stay out of their way and not want to cause issues. Looking back, I think I felt responsible because I knew Noah hadn't really chatted to them about me being around more. If he had, I'd have felt more at ease.

'It comes down to communication and respect – letting people know that you are aware of them and considering their feelings, and opening up a dialogue for all to voice their concerns,' says Emma. 'Try not to fall into the trap of trying to impress someone, be that your date or their housemates – just be yourself and find out whether this is the right set-up for you. Sometimes we worry too much about what other people think of us, and we forget to ask ourselves what we think of them.'

To respect the relationships in your house share while simultaneously carving out the time and space you need to get to know the person you're dating, you need to be considerate and communicate sensitively as you juggle the shifting priorities in your life. And when you find a balance that works, you can override some of the annoyances to focus on the perks of dating in a house share, like bonding over the hilarity of dating stories, looking out for one another, and the in-house support network.

Chapter reflections

When you look at your relationships, where does your house share sit?

Thinking about all the relationships in your life today, where do your housemates sit among them? Emma has a useful framework that can help you place them. 'Imagine a set of concentric circles,' she says. 'The relationships in your life that feel the most significant are at the centre, then the people you're closest to after that are in the ring outside that, and then your friends, and then colleagues, then a ring for your neighbours, then one for people you pass in the street. Where do your housemates sit? Perhaps your housemates make a good reality-checking stage when you're dating – checking in on how you're feeling day to day – but when it comes to who the person is or the way the relationship is unfolding, you can create a distance from their opinions.'

Ask yourself, 'Am I giving my housemates' opinions too much weight?'

A helpful sense check, if you're worrying about what your housemates are thinking or feeling about your dating habits, is to be clear about how much your housemates' opinions really matter to you. Just because they would handle a scenario differently doesn't mean you have to.

'If we're trying to create something that feels like home in a house share, let's make it the good bits of home,' says Emma. 'Unlike our last experience of home, which might have been when we were in our family of origin, power doesn't need to exist in consensus or an authority. You have the power to make your own choices – you're an independent adult, living in a house share.'

What would the dating section of your contract with your

housemates look like?

If your dating situation or relationship changes, think about how you want your housemate relationships to work and communicate that. Perhaps you're in a new relationship but want to carve out some time to be in the house share one weeknight so you can keep in touch with your housemates. 'Look at what you will bring to the relationship and what they will bring,' says Emma. 'Draw a metaphorical contract each time you feel the housemate relationships shifting, to make space for dating or a romantic relationship.' Ask yourself, 'How do I want it to look now?' Is there some crossover between your housemates' wants and needs and your own? Seeing where you're aligned or can meet in the middle, while honouring what's going on in your dating lives, is a good way to find the commonalities, so you can then establish a rhythm that works for both of you.

When it comes to sex, how can you communicate to your housemates what you're comfortable and uncomfortable with?

Perhaps you just hate talking about sex full stop, and would like total privacy, so are happy to grant your housemates this too. Perhaps a housemate bringing a one-night stand back who you've never met makes you feel anxious, and you'd really like it if your housemates would just give you a heads up when that happened. You might be nervous that your housemate's new boyfriend will start staying over more than you're happy with. Drawing on your house sharing experiences to date will help you to be clear in your mind about what you feel you can tolerate and what you can't. Then, find a way of communicating this to your housemates. Ask your housemates what they're comfortable with, too, and, together, you can find a compromise that allows each housemate to date in a way that works for every other member of the household.

How can you introduce the person you're dating to your

housemates in a clear but calm way?

Without putting too much pressure on it (because we all want to play it cool at the beginning), think of some ways that feel right to clearly communicate to your housemates this is someone you want to be able to invite over to your house share. The person you're dating will likely feel more at ease knowing that they're welcome and expected in the space. You could send a text to the group chat or, if you'd rather not announce it there, you could mention it to each housemate individually.

9. It's time

Shutting the door on a house share

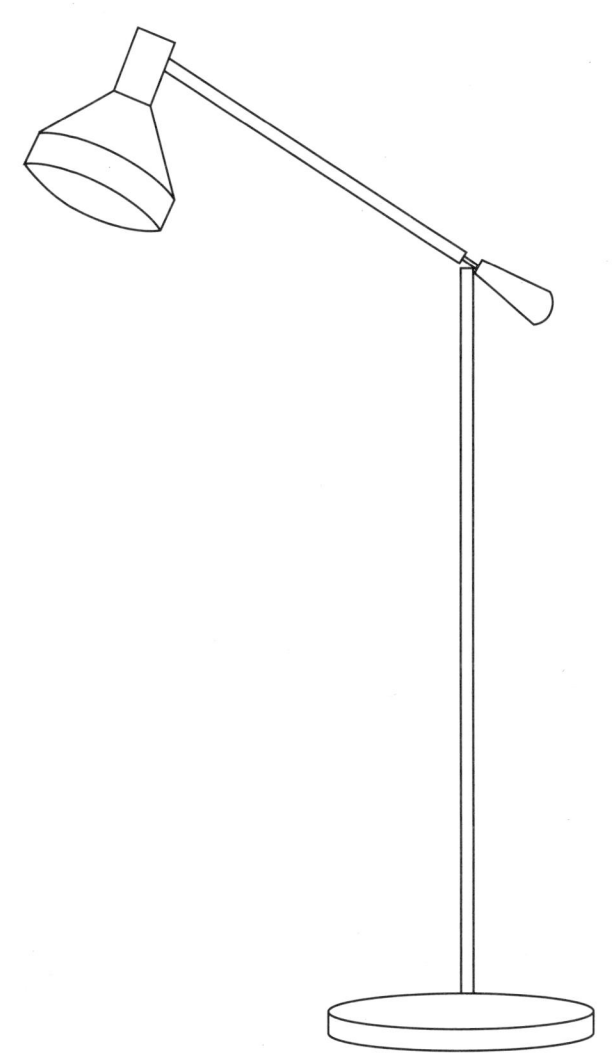

"We craft love from heartbreak, compassion
from shame, grace from disappointment,
courage from failure."
Brené Brown[1]

I have a memory of walking up the stairs to my second-floor house share in Balham, which I shared with Phoebe, Jess, and Sophie. It's dark and eerily quiet. Usually, a couple of my housemates would be around at this time of the week, performing Sunday-night rituals: making their lunches for Monday or unwinding, watching TV. As the harsh lighting flickers on in the kitchen, I spot Sophie's set of keys laid out on the worktop and that her shelf in the kitchen is bare.

The date that she's been going to depart the house share has been marked on my calendar for three months at this point. She's now left me, Phoebe, and Jess and moved in with her boyfriend. We've woken up a few steps away from each other most days for the past three years, her just the other side of the stud wall between our rooms on the top floor of our flat. Now she's moved out, the house share has changed irreversibly overnight – and, with it, our relationship as housemates.

Piles of her belongings have been appearing around the flat for weeks as she's been gathering her bits together, her presence slowly disappearing from the communal spaces. Despite the long notice period, the hole she's left behind feels vast.

We often talk about moving house as being one of the most stressful events in life.² In surveys, it's ranked as even more stressful than divorce or having a child. The upheaval that comes with moving into a new space and new area at the same time as leaving the old ones behind is a lot to deal with all at once. And, as house sharers, when you move house share or change housemates, it's not only the physical space that alters – you leave behind the people and the relationships too.

And, as more of us are living in house shares for longer than ever before, we may face this stress and upheaval more than most. The number of house sharers aged between 35 and 44 rose by 186 per cent between 2009 and 2014, reports from SpareRoom show.³ Yet, despite this rise, the physical and emotional transition that occurs when we change house shares and housemates is not generally acknowledged, let alone given any weight. Only my sisters and a few friends mark my moving into a new house share with a 'new home' card. Not considered a significant move in wider society, it's a milestone we let slip through the cracks. Perhaps if we acknowledged and celebrated leaving house shares as we do other life stages, we would be able to fully appreciate their significance and the ways they shape our lives – both when we're living in them and beyond.

Inevitable endings

Whether it's you or one of your housemates moving out to live with a partner, because of a disagreement in the house share, the landlord ending the contract, getting a promotion, which means you can afford a better place, wanting a change, wanting to explore a new neighbourhood, wanting to live with fewer people, a bigger room, a more modern space, somewhere that's got a bath... there are a huge number of reasons why a particular house share comes to an end. If we take the people I interviewed for this book as a representative group, their average age was 30 and the number of house shares they'd each lived in was five. Woven into every one of those house share moves and housemate changeovers was the ending of a life phase and the ending of a set of housemate relationships too.

Endings are an unavoidable part of house sharing. From unbearable grime to a lack of cohesion in the group to differing lifestyles, the list of valid reasons to move on is long. I left Patrick in Elephant and Castle because of the late-night antics that were keeping me up on school nights. I left East Dulwich when I'd had enough of Emma having 3am sex in the communal spaces. I left Weir Road because my friends were moving out. I left another house share where I was living with a woman much older than me because I felt that my partying was getting annoying for her. I left the second Balham house share to move in with a partner. When I left a house share, the lack of conversation and acknowledgement that things were ending resulted in complicated feelings and tension in the relationships I had with my housemates. Only once did I have honest conversations about the fact that the house share was ending and what it meant for us.

I remember how that time began. I was on my way home from work when I got a text from Lottie in the Weird Road house chat.

LOTTIE: Is everyone in tonight? Can we have a house chat? Have got some wine xx

ME: I'm on my way back now. Shall I get another bottle? Crisps?

LOTTIE: Yeah, lovely. See you in few xx

These house chats weren't unusual. Previously we covered rent going up, contract renewal, and house party plans. But when I walk in on this day, both Lottie and Sima are smiling in a knowing way that puts me on edge. Like they have something to confess.

'So, yeah, we're really sad,' says Lottie, 'but when the contract comes up in the summer, Sima and I are going to start looking to move to a smaller flat in east London. We just want to live somewhere a bit more modern and with fewer people.'

I smile and try to sound excited for them, asking about where in east London and what kind of place they're looking for. They're both a little older than me, earn more. I get it. But the news that they're leaving and putting an end to our house share stings, and I can feel my eyes fill with tears. Lottie gives me a hug and asks me what I think I'll do.

Over the next few weeks, chats about our respective next moves happen frequently and casually over quick catch-ups in the kitchen while we're all cooking dinner and longer chats on lazy weekend mornings. I share where I've looked and ideas of where I think I'll move on to, and Lottie and Sima share the flats they've been viewing. As we openly discuss our next moves, we're making plans for barbeques and gatherings in our new places. Unknowingly, we're processing the change together, readying ourselves for how our relationships will alter but agreeing that, without a doubt, we'll remain close. Initially I'd felt rejected by their decision to move on without me, but these chats helped me to reframe it.

As housemates, we need to have two conversations concurrently: one in which we deal with the practical, and one in which we address the emotional, giving space for both sets of processes to occur. So, for the first, ask, 'Can we just have a very practical chat about dates I'm moving out or tying up the bills?' This leaves room for the second, more emotionally charged conversations about how your relationships will change to occur separately.

Amelia Rees, 31, lives in Highbury, north London. She has lived in five house shares in total, in Surrey, London, and Bristol. She has had experience of being the housemate who left as well as the one who stayed behind when her housemate went, and reflects that the endings were not really dealt with head on.

'For me, the endings of house shares have always felt a bit

messy,' she says. 'When I left a house share in Bristol, where I'd been one of the original tenants and was in charge of all the bills and the logins, it opened a can of worms because the others decided they didn't want to stay either. So then I had six years' worth of stuff to clear out of the house where 12 housemates had lived during that time. I had to contact the ex-housemates and ask for information on where bits of furniture had gone or if they had proof of permission to make alterations to the house. It was one of the most stressful times I've had house sharing. But, on an emotional level, because I was the one leaving, I was also focused on what was coming next and thinking about the place I was moving to.'

Fractious house share endings are, like so many other aspects of house sharing, a symptom of us not having universally accepted tools or paths to follow through this life stage. There are socially acceptable phrases and conversations that we know to use when dealing with change in a romantic relationship or a job, and we need these for house sharers too.

Two sides of the same coin

At the end of a romantic relationship, there's usually an 'ender' and an 'endee'. Most of us will know that it's easier for the ender to process this change as they made the decision and have a clear reason for moving on. The person doing the breaking up is usually a step ahead in the grieving process, as clinical psychologist Peter Kanaris explains in an article in *The Psychologist*:[4] 'The person that initiates the break-up has already processed many of the thoughts and the feelings related to that kind of separation and has looked forward to some extent – what is coming up in life, there may be a new relationship or a new lifestyle that is emerging.'

There are some similarities here with house shares. While one housemate might be moving out and looking forward to a positive change in their life – particularly if they're moving in with a partner – the other might be staying in the house share and having complicated feelings about a period of their life they were enjoying and wanted to continue enjoying. Without careful recalibration of our relationships, it's hard not to reduce ourselves to 'the one who's moving forward' and 'the one who's being left behind'.

As the housemate leaving a house share, you're playing a proactive role, thinking of the bigger picture of your life and seeing how leaving a house share is the first step towards achieving it. When you're the housemate being left behind, you're reacting to this new situation – you have to find a way to deal with something that is beyond your control and, as a direct result of someone else's choices, there's a lot of recalibrating to do.

Nicolette Wilding, 32, is a writer from Hackney. She struggled to find the words when a house share she lived in for two years with her best friend of 20 years came to an end. She describes how, when her friend started a new relationship, she began to have complicated feelings about ending their time living together. 'When my housemate got into a relationship, I sort of knew that it would potentially directly impact my own future living situation. There's a very high potential that it can change quickly because, now, if she really likes him, it's a real possibility that she might end up moving in with him or marrying him.'

Nicolette's housemate was in a relationship that was becoming more serious. For another housemate, there might be a new job they've been interviewing for over a few months. Similar to an ender's position in a romantic relationship, they will have had time to process the change that's happening and leaving a house share is just one part of their new beginning. Like an endee, the person being left in a house share has to deal with the outcome of a choice that wasn't theirs and has had less time to process it. Also, whereas the housemate who has made the decision to leave because it fits in with their plan for their near future, often, for the person being left, it doesn't fit in with their plans for their near future quite so neatly.

The two differing positions the housemates are in – one proactive and one reactive – make for a tricky conversation between them, as Nicolette describes. 'I would never say, "Because that lovely thing is happening in your life, I feel a pressure to make it happen in my life or I'm going to be alone." It doesn't feel like a rational thing that I can even really address or bring up with my housemate. Even if that is how the kicking child inside me feels. Instead, I try to think of what I'd want if it was me in that position.

'It has the potential to put a wedge in your relationship where it never was before. I think underneath it all is the way housing is set up, and the fact that our pay doesn't afford us the option to have a space of our own, so there's a lot of pressure on housemates to keep a good thing going. It has an impact on your friendship dynamic but also literally where you can live. I do think there's a bit of an inescapable feeling of, "Oh, OK. Well, that ends that fun."'

Being the endee – the one left behind

Making sense of the feelings that occur when a housemate moves is complex. I knew I'd stay in touch with Sophie when she left the house share in Balham, but living there without her by my side had a profound impact on my day-to-day life. I didn't have the language to explain this loss to anyone else. I missed her, but didn't feel like I had the right to feel her departure so deeply.

My connection with Sophie had been a slow burn. We met for the first time when I moved in and, in the initial 12 months, we formed a steady but strong relationship – a low-maintenance connection that felt secure and gentle. She liked routine and her mornings followed a regular pattern, whereas every morning looked different for me. The steady rhythm of her morning rituals became a comforting backing track to my chaotic lack of them.

When the day of Sophie's moving out arrived, I decided to go out to meet a friend. The house is alive with people carrying boxes; I want to give Sophie some space. I also want to protect myself from the sadness I feel about watching the housemate I've shared so much with disappear from my life, box by box. By the time I arrive home again, everything's still. Sophie has gone.

I walk into her room. It still smells of her perfume and her washing powder, but there's no sign she's ever lived there. I feel the emptiness of it. Our lives, wherever they go next, will never come back here, to this house share, to a time when our daily routines were so respectfully and beautifully intertwined.

I chatted to the other two housemates, but the conversation was stilted, a little awkward, and it turned into a practical conversation about trying to find a replacement. None of us really knew how to talk properly about the impact Sophie leaving the house share had on us.

In his book *Necessary Endings*, clinical psychologist Dr Henry Cloud talks about how proactively processing endings is part of moving forward. He writes, 'If you have emotional or other energy invested in something, when you pull that out, and let go, you are going to feel it. For every action there is an equal and opposite reaction, so if you make a move to end something you are invested in, there will be an impact. And if you do not deal with those feelings, you are going to do some funny things to get around them.'[5] I wasn't proactive. I left the flat the morning of Sophie's departure to avoid feeling the sadness, unable to open a conversation about how sad I really was to see her go. Also, partly, I didn't want to dampen the mood when Sophie herself was so excited about the next phase in her life.

There is a special type of stress house sharers are subjected to more than most: the need to react to ever-changing circumstances in our homes. We're forced to find ways to deal with the fact that we're about to lose our home as we know it, whether it's because a housemate is moving on or the landlord is selling the place or wants to do it up.

It's not always just the people who are leaving that you grieve, it's the physical space too. Anyone who has left a home behind – a childhood home, a first flat, or your fifth house share – will know how emotional it can be to extract yourself from the walls that, for the time you were living there, witnessed and held so much. From childhood memories to messy parties to it being our first home with a partner, our homes have a way of physically holding whatever took place there. They become important characters in our lives.

Sometimes when we're house sharing, we have to move because of something that's beyond our control and, in a similar way to being the endee in a romantic relationship, having to leave a home because of a decision someone else has made can make it harder to process than if we were the ender. Instead of being a choice that you've pondered and weighed up, it is a situation not of your making that you must react to. You have no choice but to divert your path if all your housemates are moving on or your landlord wants to sell up.

When I lived in the Weir Road flat, I remember feeling completely at sea when Lottie and Sima told me that they wanted to move to a different part of the city and to a smaller flat. Even though they explained the practical reasons – they'd be closer to work and Sima's boyfriend lived closer to there – it did feel like a horrible rejection. We had, until then, been sailing along as a group and, now, they were choosing to break that up. Because it wasn't my decision, I had to take some time to process the impact that was going to have on me and what my next step looked like.

'The time I was the housemate being left, I was really, really upset,' remembers Amelia, who now lives in Highbury. 'We had formed such a tight bond by then. We'd sit in the lounge together and eat, watch *Love Island*, play rounders together on a Tuesday evening after work. So when they told me they were leaving, I was like, "Oh my gosh, wow. What am I going to do?"'

I ask psychotherapist Alex Iga Golabeck how she might approach supporting someone in a house share who is having to deal with a change in their living circumstance that feels very out of their hands. She says the first step is facing up to the lack of control you're feeling. 'A sense of powerlessness breeds problems of its own, so it's important to be aware of it. Even just reminding yourself, "This is uncomfortable because it's not within my control."' She adds, 'As humans, we're not supposed to feel powerless or overwhelmed for too long and, if you do, it can cause problematic behaviours. You might notice yourself becoming increasingly obsessed with social media or overworking. That's you chasing something that gives you a sense of control.

'The truth is, you have some element of control, but you might just not feel like you do. Yes, circumstances have changed and you might have to move out of the house share you're currently in. Your choice and your power lies in what you do next. Will you stay and find a replacement? Or will you move on? You have the power because you have the opportunity to look at the circumstances in front of you and say, "That's not good enough for me, so I will move." Or whatever it is you decide.'

The other thing Alex thinks it is important to consider is the merits of impermanence that you're benefiting from. It might be that, right now, you're the one having to divert your path because of a housemate leaving or a landlord selling the place but, one day soon, it will be you who is benefiting from the impermanence of the set-up. 'You can look at the impermanence as a hopeful thing, too, because when it doesn't work for you any more, you can also move on.'

Being the ender – the one departing

As we've seen, for the housemate leaving, there's usually a meaningful reason they've come to terms with that helps them to make sense of the ending. Sophie, the first of the original set of housemates to leave our Balham house share, definitely seemed to be approaching her departure with excitement, understandably looking forward to this new stage in her life.

A year after Sophie moved out, I followed in her footsteps and moved in with my partner, leaving that Balham house share behind. I experienced a different form of the same grief I'd felt when Sophie left – the other side of that coin. I was so excited about having our own space that I didn't allow myself to truly acknowledge how much I was leaving behind. It was only six months into living in the new flat with my partner that I realised how much I missed the intimate and nourishing connections arising from living alongside the women I had house shared with. At that point, not knowing my path would take me back to a house share in the future, I didn't think I'd ever have that again.

The contract we sign when we move in to a house share in no way reflects the connections and relationships that we build while we live there, which creates a tension. On the one hand, yes, our legal responsibility stops when we give our notice and, perhaps, find a replacement housemate. We have the right to terminate the contract and cease our involvement in that house share by simply sending an email. But this in no way honours the family of sorts we might have created there. Yet that contract is why so many house sharers deny themselves the right to feel the emotions of the situation and process the ending, rationalising it was always going to happen and they don't have any claims over their housemates or the relationships they built in the house share.

You may recall an idea mentioned in Chapter 3 in relation to cohabiting – that it is better to decide to, not slide into it, to make deliberate choices rather than be led by circumstances – and explored as applying to house shares by being self-aware when moving in with friends. It can be helpful in the context of departing a house share too. If we pay attention to the changes in the relationships when a house share ends and the emotions that result – as Lottie, Sima, and I did when we left Weir Road – then we can make smooth transitions that feel healthy. We can learn from each house share, and we can feel excited about the prospect of living somewhere new as well as fully celebrate the time in the house share we're leaving behind.

Doing endings better

Amelia reflects on how the last house share she left ended. 'I didn't do a very good job of closing that chapter of my life properly, but I think it's because I felt I didn't really have a claim on my housemates as people. They're not officially friends or partners. You live in the house share alongside one another and you're bumbling along but, in the background, you always know that at some point it will end.

'I felt the same when another house share ended, where I'd been living with a woman who, over the three years, had become a really good friend. She'd met a partner and so I was moving out. The conversation we had about ending the house share was a bit fraught. I think it was just because neither of us knew how to talk about it. We're really close friends now, but it took some work to get it back on track.'

When I didn't properly process Sophie leaving the Balham house share, it left me with residual feelings that had a negative impact on how I felt towards the next housemate to take her room. Without Sophie, the dynamic in the house had shifted. I missed the closeness that we had shared. Living side by side on the top floor together, I would spend more time with her than with the others. When a new housemate, Jen, moved in to live in the room next to mine, I assumed that the same thing would happen as before and so the closeness I'd shared with Sophie would return to the house share with her arrival. In actual fact, Jen grew closer to Phoebe, one of my other housemates, and so my sense of loss deepened rather than went away. Similar to how some people behave in rebound scenarios in romantic relationships, I was masking my sadness that Sophie had left and, as a result, struggling to make meaningful and genuine connections with the new housemate and new house share dynamic.

As well as reflecting on the specific situation, being proactive about processing the feeling of loss when a housemate leaves can be powerful. In a study by researchers at the University of Colorado,[6] participants going through break-ups and dealing with rejection were given a nasal spray. Half the participants were told that the spray would improve the symptoms of their emotional pain and the other half were told it was a placebo saline solution. Those who thought they'd been given something to help reduce their emotional pain reported an improvement and images of their brains showed increased activity in areas that regulate emotion and reduced activity in areas that feel pain. The takeaway is that, if you feel like something you're doing is directly helping you to deal with feelings of loss – whether it's keeping in touch with a housemate who's moved out, chatting with friends, journaling about the transition, going for walks to help process the feelings, or spraying saline up your nose – it will help.

For Amelia, many of her former housemates remain good friends of hers today. She talks about that transition from housemate to friend. 'There were some house shares I left and we had a house dinner to mark the occasion but, beyond that, the conversations were very practical and there was no love lost. We moved on and lost touch. But when there have been housemates I've been close with, it has been a case of creating space for them in my life in the same way you'd see other friends you don't live with. And, actually, engaging with their social media is quite powerful. You sort of transfer that low-level daily contact and you're aware of what they're up to without it being a super-intense friendship. There's so much you're used to getting updates on when they get home from work when you live together, and it's about finding a way of keeping in touch that's sustainable for both of you beyond your house share.'

When we are invested in our house share or our housemates – even if it's the kind of low-level investment that I felt sharing a home with Sophie – the relationships we've formed there are going to be altered when someone leaves. Either we decide that it's a connection we will let go or it's one we will invest in and make time for beyond the house share. Like a notice period on a job, there's usually a long goodbye in a house share before the contract is officially up or someone moves out. It's a time we can use to end things properly, so we have the energy to pour into what happens next, which might include a new style of relationship with a former housemate.

A living loss

The loss of a housemate relationship – whether they're the one moving out or you are – is a type of 'living loss', which is the term used for a significant change that alters our day-to-day life and leaves us grieving a former existence or relationship. It's loss, but not a finite loss – the housemate and group of housemates haven't died – but the once physical circumstances of and how you once connected with one another have.

Dr Becca Bland is a specialist in estrangement in family relationships, coaching people to understand the complexities of living loss and move forward in their lives. I ask her to explain what makes living loss different from grief. 'A living loss is a complex grief,' she says. 'It's a sense that you're losing someone but it's hard to process because they're still living and breathing. When someone we love dies, we have a very firm ending to a relationship, because we get a piece of paper, a reason why they're not with us, and a finality ritual, often a funeral. There's more understanding in society that losing people to death is very difficult.

'With a living loss, we lose people because they've moved on. They could be housemates, ex-partners, or friends. They're still living but we lose them from our lives, and it leaves a significant void where physical presence used to be. We may feel distance and space in terms of communication, but the cords of the relationship still exist. We know that one day we may meet that person again, we may hear about their lives from others, or see them on social media. So, we're left negotiating with ourselves as we face that lingering feeling that a relationship with that person could exist but isn't actually happening any more. It's a loss and a grief and often it's complex to navigate, especially if there's been conflict.'

Becca identifies five stages of grief when someone is dealing with a living loss. One is disassociation, which is when you create mental distance from the feelings that are occurring and might feel quite detached from what's happening around you as a result. 'If we are the one disassociating from a relationship, we get away from the stimulus that is causing us to feel pain and difficulty,' she says.

I've definitely had these feelings in house shares when I've known I was about to depart, a housemate was leaving, or the house share was coming to an end. Instead of facing up to the sadness, I ignored it, pretending it wasn't happening, and filled my time with looking to the future. It's why, on the day Sophie left, I went out to meet a friend.

Another stage in the grieving process is feeling anger and sadness – and these might be misdirected anger and sadness. So perhaps it's manifesting in feeling frustrated about the process of finding another house share or housemate. The next stage is letting go, when we distinguish what we can and can't control. Feeling strength is the stage that follows, which involves seeing what the house share you're leaving has given you that is positive. The final stage is finding peace, achieving a sense of acceptance as you move forwards.

'When I work in my coaching sessions with people facing a living loss, we firstly decide on an objective of where they want to get to,' says Becca. 'We notice and look at the thoughts and feelings getting in their way. I'd help them look at what they can and can't control, to reframe unhelpful thoughts, address the situation and help them feel more empowered.'

This is a helpful framework to apply to the ending of a house share. First, decide what it is you'd like out of the relationships with your soon-to-be-former housemates in the future, then observe what's stopping you from making that happen, and whether it's something in your power to control or not. So, if the housemate who's departing doesn't seem to have the same desire to keep in touch as you, that is out of your control, and you'd be better focusing instead on finding a way of processing the time you've had together.

Rituals

Becca recalls a time when she was house sharing and a housemate moved out. 'I remember being incredibly hurt in the last house share I lived in with one other woman,' she says.

'We had become really close friends – we shared so much of our lives and I was always a stakeholder in her romantic relationships. Then, she very suddenly decided to move abroad. She immediately started packing and focusing on logistics, and there was just such an emotional piece missing from her. There was a real loss there for me, but it just didn't seem like she really felt it. It felt uneasy and hurtful, like I was being abandoned.

'When you're house sharing, there's a curious dance that goes on where you're not really like family, but you are family because you're sharing a space and an energy, a whole lifestyle together. That's very bonding. It's very close; it can often be really supportive. They're your closest people who you see every day. So when you move away from that, how do you negotiate that relationship? To you, it might have a lot of meaning, but that might not be the case for your housemate. Perhaps to them you are just someone who they shared a house with. There's this lingering emotional cord that formed between you and, while you might not have communication or contact, you still feel that, even when you've stopped living together.

'Looking back, and with my coach head on, what would have been better is if we'd had some kind of ritual to honour what we'd shared. Marking the ending of something is really powerful. Whether it's cooking together, going out for a meal, or throwing a party, create a space where you can reflect on why that period of your life has been so special.'

By marking the end of an era with a difficult but cathartic conversation or a celebration to mark what's come before, we give ourselves the space to fully embrace all that's to come by either tying up the cords of our relationships or nurturing them so that they thrive beyond the house share.

When Nicolette, the writer from Hackney, left the house share she was living in with her best friend, marking the end of the house share with a ritual and some reflection felt really powerful for her. 'As we were both packing down the flat and looking at all the things we'd accumulated together, we just naturally started reminiscing about the years we'd lived there together. Then we cooked a full roast to mark the end of our time there. It felt really sentimental and like a way of acknowledging the family we'd made between us two. We had three courses, champagne, and a selection of desserts because we both love dessert. We talked about where we were in our lives compared with when we first moved in, and all the things that had happened – both good and bad. It felt really nice to acknowledge that that period of time was ending because it was a significant time. She's my best friend. We have changed a lot in the time we lived together but, through all the obstacles, we did always manage to keep our relationship strong.'

My time at Weir Road, where I lived with Sima and Lottie, ended as it had begun: with a big house party. Instead of being a guest, cautiously approaching the doorway, I was a host, holding open the door to the faces that were familiar to me now after two years of living there. Sima bought multicoloured helium balloons that spelled out 'WEIR'. They wafted prominently in the living room, in between a set of massive speakers and a table that was set up for beer pong. Lottie made the lethal punch that she'd become well known for. Eric the rabbit was relocated in her bedroom. I went around trying to hide stuff that we wouldn't want people to use to drink out of – or be sick in.

The night unfolded, following the same familiar pattern of the house parties that had come before it: sober mingling at the drinks station in our tiny galley kitchen; deep, meaningful – and drunken – conversations on the landing and stairs; people sneaking into bedrooms they weren't meant to; a group of 20-somethings sitting down crossed-legged on the floor playing drinking games. The party was a ritual that ended our time there perfectly and, simultaneously, worked as a launch party of sorts for what came next. We had alcohol-fuelled chats about how much we were going to miss one another and made immediate plans to continue the fun we'd had there.

Our homes and, by extension, our house shares have a profound impact on our lives and emotional health. Social psychologist Dr Sandra Wheatley explains that this is because it's an ingrained system which has worked for humans since the beginning of time. 'On a very basic level, our homes satisfy a very primal need for shelter,' she says. 'Over a lifetime, our homes imprint on our memories because, for most of us, they're places we've felt safe enough to develop. If you think back to when you were growing up, maybe you can still smell the carpet, imagine the texture of the curtains, the shape of the door handles. When you're house sharing, the development looks different but still mimics this evolutionary need to live alongside others who give us that feeling of safety we need to develop.'

Still today, 10 years after moving on from that flat share, Lottie, Sima, and I, plus others from that Weir Road house party gang, holiday together. I still remember exactly how each of them takes their morning cups of tea, their individual dietary requirements, who snores, and who makes retching noises when they brush their teeth. Maybe you remember tiny details about your housemates and house shares that you've departed. For me, those intimate details acquired from the years living together make it easy to snap right back into the group and continue the fun we started in that house share on Weir Road.

'The memories we make in our houses mean we form a strong connection with that place,' says Sandra. 'Leaving them is emotional, but it is a natural evolution. It's important not to shy away from it, but the truth is, when you've bonded well with your housemates and made happy memories inside a house share, it's not really the end. It's a progression of those connections.'

Chapter reflections

How can you make room for the practical *and* the emotional when leaving a house share?

It can be helpful just to say to your housemates, 'There are a lot of logistics involved with me moving on and I'll do what I can to make it as smooth as possible. But I'm also personally really sad to be leaving our house share and I'd like to find a way to mark the end of our time living together.' If you can do this early on in the discussions, it'll open the floor for your other housemates to share their feelings and reflect on their time living with you too.

If you're staying and your housemate is leaving, can you find a way to open up a conversation to share your feelings?

It might go something like this: 'I'm really excited about your next move. But, at the same time, I'm sad that our time living together is coming to an end. I wonder if we can mark it with a leaving dinner or drinks? I'd love to reminisce about our time living together before you go.'

Can you coach yourself through the ending?

Can you use the format of Dr Becca Bland's coaching session to shape your own thoughts about leaving or being left in a house share? What would you like the relationship with your soon-to-be former housemate to be? What are the thoughts and feelings getting in the way of achieving that? What parts of it can you control? What can't you control? How can you reframe your approach?

What rituals would help to mark the ending and, if you want to, begin the next phase of your friendship?

Rituals help us to acknowledge the change happening to our living situation and to look back on the happy times we've had together. Making sure you have no regrets is a helpful part of being able to look forwards. It might be dinner, a night out, a walk and a coffee... Whatever you choose, make sure it's something that reflects the essence of your time together. Take photos and videos, write cards, and make memories. And, if you feel able to, ask each housemate to answer some reflective questions. What worked? What are you grateful for? What do you appreciate about one another? What will you miss? How will you stay in touch in the future? What is it that made the house share experience truly special and something that you will carry with you for ever?

Conclusion

We often hear about how people's lives are shaped by romantic relationships – in day-to-day life, novels, and romantic comedies. How, when two people partner up, they come together and create a rhythm to their lives, one shaped by shared interests, connection, love, and care. When we talk about finding a romantic partner, we look for someone who magnifies the good parts of our character, shines a light on the challenging parts of our personality, and makes us want to be a better person. We hear, too, about how partners create a life and grow together.

When I look back at the past 10 years of my life, it's my housemates who have shaped my character more than any romantic partner. During my 20s, it was my housemates who encouraged me to grow – sometimes in ways that forced me to face uncomfortable truths about myself; sometimes in unexpectedly wonderful ways. I met people, learned about others' lives, challenged my own preconceptions, looked at things from new perspectives, and tried things I wouldn't have done otherwise.

I rehearsed work presentations in front of housemates, knocked on their doors at midnight needing an interview-appropriate jacket for the next morning, and aired work stresses while frying a salmon fillet to these people who knew what it was like to be a woman in the workplace and would help me to find solutions. I celebrated leaving bad jobs and finding new ones with them. We bonded over the unavoidable despair of modern dating, shared in the excitement of meeting someone new, and metaphorically held one another's hands through the anxieties that come with those early stages of new relationships. I've learned to cook things I'd otherwise never have thought to cook. We planned day trips to the coast, did our toiletry shopping together on Saturday mornings, pooled period supplies, left little pick-me-up notes and chocolates, bought flowers for each other's bedrooms. These small, enforced acts of affection only possible when you live together become the foundations of true intimacy.

With that closeness comes an unspoken commitment. One that sometimes feels confusing and frustrating. Are my expectations of my housemates too high when, technically, we only share names on a tenancy agreement? Is it OK to feel so affected by the tensions between us? They're just housemates, it is just a temporary arrangement. These are questions that I've asked and heard others asking when I interviewed them for this book. Despite a decade of living in house shares, I never realised quite how many of us feel silly and ashamed of just how much of an impact our house share and housemate relationships have on our day-to-day lives and emotional wellbeing.

It's a result, I think, of society not holding these relationships in as high esteem as we do romantic relationships. If, in 10 years' time, the self-help bookshelves come to be filled with 'how to live in house share' books, we will be in a place where house sharing relationships are just as much part of social discourse as modern dating. In that future, perhaps it will be as normal to talk about housemate break-ups as it is now to reference couples breaking up.

The truth is, the people we live with shape our lives in ways that we can neither control nor predict. Sometimes it's for the better, sometimes it's less than ideal. How we work with this is the only thing we can control. Moving out is always an option but, as I know all too well, doing this frequently is discombobulating and unsettling, and usually happens at a time in your life when you are craving some level of stability.

I interviewed the psychologists and other experts whose words you have been reading in this book during the first few months in a new house share – my eighth in London. This meant that I put their advice into practice and tried to do things differently and better this time. I felt myself enter into my house sharing life properly, have those difficult conversations, invest an appropriate amount of emotion, and ask for what I need to make the house share feel like home. When I started dating again, I felt so much more prepared for the conversations about having someone over.

And, when irritations arise, I allow myself to feel them, no longer brushing them off as 'just some temporary frustration'. I think about what might be going on for my housemate and gently open conversations with her, even when they are the sweaty-palmed kind. I have felt more invested and more at peace here as a result.

I have also realised how knowing more about myself – what my reflex in response to conflict is and my attachment style – helps me to frame what's occurring for me. These are skills we can hone in house shares but, ultimately, they are skills that then stay with us for life. They help us to find our way through friendships, working relationships, and romantic partnerships. The lessons I have learned from living with a wide range of different people and personality types have, I think, made me a more understanding and empathetic person than I would ever have been otherwise.

House shares can be intense. Exploring the issues that arise – from living with friends to dating in a house share to experiencing a living loss when a house share ends – I have delved into group psychology, couples therapy, and attachment theory. On many occasions, the psychologists and other experts I interviewed were clearly perplexed by situations I described to them – by the intensity, variety of characters, and lack of guidance we face in house shares. All of this playing out under one – usually modest – roof. And if you're in a house share, you'll know that you're navigating it all on a daily basis.

When we understand how to negotiate the twists and turns in a house share well, something bigger shifts. What we are doing is about more than just staying sane in a house share. It gives rise to a hope and a confidence that extends beyond the four walls of your house of multiple occupancy. You see how powerful it can be to tune in to what it takes to live harmoniously alongside other humans who, although they might not have the same dreams, vulnerabilities, and hygiene levels as us, nonetheless offer us connection, support, and – for a time – a feeling that we are home.

Acknowledgements

Thank you, Megan, for being the calm and collected agent you are, and for being excited about this book from the very beginning. To my editor, Elizabeth, for your encouragement, kindness, and editorial wisdom. I'm so fortunate to have worked with you on my first book.

To Morgan Rees, Penny Wincer, Adi Bloom, Jonny Cooper, Liz Beardsell, and Charlotte Moore – writers, editors, and sounding boards – thank you for your support and giving me the space to get this book off the ground.

To all the women (and the one man) who welcomed me into their homes and gave me a window into their house sharing life. Every conversation reminded me why I started writing this book. Thank you for trusting me with your feelings and your stories.

To the psychologists and other experts I interviewed, who gave me their time and advice. Thank you for responding so thoughtfully to my questions and giving me robust and heartfelt answers. I know your words will help so many.

To all the housemates I have lived with in my eight house shares. Thank you for showing me how special living together can be and for sharing your lives with me for the time we were under the same roof – I know that I'll always look back on these years and smile.

To Lucy and Laura, for constructing and reconstructing furniture with me, rocking up at various kitchen tables across London with wine, a listening ear, and lots to laugh about, and housing me (and my always overflowing bags) in your spare rooms.

To 'the girls' – my sisters, Emily and Beth – my very first housemates. What fun we had. Thank you for picking up the phone at all hours and teaching me from a young age that it's not

OK to wear other people's clothes. To Edward, Margot, Henry, Wilfred, Polly, and Olive, thank you for the endless cuddles and never failing to make me laugh out loud – I love you all so much.

And to my mum, for always believing in me and my writing, and showing me how powerful it is when you do the little things that make you feel at home.

Notes

1. A room of her own

1 Virginia Woolf, *A Room of One's Own* (London: Penguin Classics, 2020), p. 76.

2 Based on an estimated 497,000 houses in multiple occupation (HMOs) in England and Wales at the end of March 2018. An HMO is defined as having at least three tenants. See Wendy Wilson and Hannah Cromarty, 'Houses in multiple occupation (HMOs) England and Wales', Briefing Paper Number 0708, House of Commons Library, 30 September 2019, available at: https://researchbriefings.files.parliament.uk/documents/SN00708/SN00708.pdf (accessed July 2024).

3 Catherine Reed, '19 intriguing roommate statistics: 2022', Flex, 30 May 2022, available at: https://getflex.com/blog/roommate-statistics/#:~:text=In%20the%20United%20States%2C%2031.9,in%20a%20housemate%2Dstyle%20situation (accessed July 2024).

4 Hilary Osborne, 'Generation rent: The housing ladder starts to collapse for the under-40s', *The Guardian,* 22 July 2015, available at: www.theguardian.com/money/2015/jul/22/pwc-report-generation-rent-to-grow-over-next-decade (accessed July 2024).

5 Osborne, 'Generation rent'.

6 Girlguiding, 'Girls' attitudes survey 2023: Girls' lives over 15 years', Girlguiding, 2023 available at: www.girlguiding.org.uk/globalassets/docs-and-resources/research-and-campaigns/girls-attitudes-summary.pdf (accessed July 2024).

7 Homeward Legal, 'UK house prices treble in 20 years', Homeward Legal, 2 January 2020, available at: www.homewardlegal.co.uk/news/post/uk-house-prices-treble-in-20-

years#:~:text=the%2021st%20century.-,Analysis%20by%20
the%20Halifax%20has%20revealed%20that%20the%20
average%20price,239%20percent%20since%20the%20
millennium (accessed July 2024).

8 Toby Helm and Jamie Doward, 'UK housing crisis: Four in
10 renters fear they will never own a home', *The Guardian,*
30 April 2016, available at: www.theguardian.com/society
/2016/apr/30/uk-throes-of--housing-crisis (accessed July 2024).

9 Matt Hutchinson, 'Demand for rooms surges', SpareRoom blog,
30 September 2021, available at: https://blog.spareroom.co.uk/
demand-for-rooms-surges (accessed July 2024).

10 Rozi Jones, 'Income to house price ratio more than doubles
since the 70s', Financial Reporter, 5 July 2023, available at:
www.financialreporter.co.uk/income-to-house-price-ratio-
more-than-doubles-since-the-70s.html#:~:text=Although%20
the%20average%20home%20may,70s%20required%204.1%20
times%20income (accessed July 2024).

11 Aimee North, 'UK House Price Index: July 2023', Office for
National Statistics (ONS), 20 September 2023, available at:
www.ons.gov.uk/economy/inflationandpriceindices/bulletins/
housepriceindex/july2023#:~:text=1.,recent%20peak%20in%20
November%202022 (accessed July 2024).

12 Statista, 'Median annual earning for full-time employees in
the United Kingdom from 1999 to 2023, by gender',
Statista, November 2023, available at: www.statista.com/
statistics/802209/full-time-annual-salary-in-the-uk-by-gender
(accessed July 2024).

13 Aimee North, 'UK House Price Index: June 2023', ONS,
16 August 2023, available at: www.ons.gov.uk/economy/
inflationandpriceindices/bulletins/housepriceindex/june2023
(accessed July 2024).

14 Lucy Buckland, 'First-time buyers now need a £65,000
deposit to get on the property ladder', MailOnline, 17 September
2011, available at: www.dailymail.co.uk/news/article-2038509/

Housing-crisis-looms-time-buyers-average-deposit-soars-65-000.html (accessed July 2024).

15 Statista, 'Median annual earning for full-time employees in the United Kingdom from 1999 to 2023, by gender'.

16 Joe Seydl, 'When will the crisis in US housing affordability end – and how?', J. P. Morgan, 14 November 2023, available at: https://privatebank.jpmorgan.com/nam/en/insights/markets-and-investing/ideas-and-insights/when-will-the-crisis-in-US-housing-affordability-end-and-how#:~:text=U.S.%20home%20prices%20are%20currently,about%2040%25%20during%20the%20pandemic.&text=Sales%20of%20existing%20homes%20are,after%20the%20global%20financial%20crisis (accessed July 2024).

17 Generation Rent, 'Saving for a mortgage deposit now takes a decade', Generation Rent, 3 July 2023, available at: www.generationrent.org/2023/07/03/saving-for-a-mortgage-deposit-now-takes-a-decade/#:~:text=Higher%20rents%20and%20house%20prices,to%20save%20for%20a%20deposit (accessed July 2024).

18 Buckland, 'First-time buyers now need a £65,000 deposit to get on the property ladder'.

19 David Burrows, 'Average homebuyer needs two years of earnings to cover deposit', Mortgage Strategy, 19 September 2023, available at: www.mortgagestrategy.co.uk/news/average-homebuyer-needs-two-years-of-earnings-to-cover-deposit (accessed July 2024).

20 Suban Abdulla, 'Cost of living crisis: Women hit harder by rents than men', Yahoo!Finance, 11 February 2022, available at: https://uk.finance.yahoo.com/news/cost-of-living-crisis-women-hit-harder-than-men-rent-energy-bills-national-insurance-000138020.html#:~:text=New%20data%20by%20SpareRoom%20shows,looming%20national%20insurance%20tax%20hike.&text=The%20flatshare%20site%20says%20over,gap%20between%20men%20and%20women (accessed July 2024).

21 Charlotte Duok, 'Pay gap, caring and confidence: Why is it still so much harder for women to buy in London than men?', *The Standard,* 24 October 2023, available at: www.standard.co.uk/ homesandproperty/property-news/property-gender-pay-gap-the-divide-in-the-housing-market-b1065397. html#:~:text=Unsurprisingly%2C%20then%2C%20women%20 account%20for,get%20on%20the%20property%20ladder (accessed July 2024).

22 ABC Finance, 'The truth behind generation rent', ABC Finance blog, n.d., available at: https://abcfinance.co.uk/blog/ generation-rent-study (accessed July 2024).

23 UK Women's Budget Group, 'Housing and gender: A pre-budget briefing from the Women's Budget Group', UK Women's Budget Group, March 2020, available at: https://wbg. org.uk/wp-content/uploads/2020/02/final-housing-2020.pdf (accessed July 2024).

24 Duok, 'Pay gap, caring and confidence'.

25 Gail Izat, 'Cost-of-living crisis has hit women harder than men, says report', Reward and Employee Benefits Association (REBA), available at: https://reba.global/resource/how-the-cost-of-living-crisis-has-affected-financial-inequality-standard-life-report.html#:~:text=The%20ongoing%20economic%20 uncertainty%20appears,finding%20their%20financial%20 situation%20difficult (accessed July 2024).

26 Eileen Patten and Kim Parker, 'A gender reversal on career aspirations: Young women now top young men in valuing a high-paying career', Pew Research Center, 19 April 2012, available at: www.pewresearch.org/socialtrends /2012/04/19/ a-gender-reversal-on-career-aspirations (accessed July 2024).

27 UN Women, 'Everything you need to know about pushing for pay equity', UN Women, 22 February 2024, available at: www. unwomen.org/en/news/stories/2020/9/explainer-everything-you-need-to-know-about-equal-pay (accessed July 2024).

28 UN Women, 'Equal pay for work of equal value', UN Women, n.d., available at: www.unwomen.org/en/news/in-focus/csw61/equal-pay (accessed July 2024).

29 Ceri Parker, 'It's official: Women work nearly an hour longer than men every day', World Economic Forum, available at: www.weforum.org/agenda/2017/06/its-official-women-work-nearly-an-hour-longer-than-men-every-day (accessed July 2024).

30 Vicky Spratt, 'I'm 34 and I have a good job – why am I still stuck in a houseshare?', Grazia, 27 February 2019, available at: https://graziadaily.co.uk/life/real-life/housing-crises-generation-rent-flatsharing (accessed July 2024).

31 Becky Dickinson, 'Middle-aged – but having to share a flat with strangers: It's a symptom of our bonkers property market, the high-earning professional women living like students', MailOnline, 11 November 2015, available at: www.dailymail.co.uk/femail/article-3314369/Middle-aged-having-share-flat-strangers-s-symptom-bonkers-property-market-high-earning-professional-women-living-like-students.html (accessed July 2024).

32 Sadhbh O'Sullivan, 'It's not just you – house sharing actually makes you miserable', Refinery29, 13 October 2023, available at: www.refinery29.com/en-gb/house-sharing-mental-health-impact (accessed July 2024).

33 ABC Finance, 'The truth behind generation rent'.

34 Relate, '"Milestone anxiety" on the rise among millennials and Gen Z', Relate, n.d., available at: www.relate.org.uk/get-help/milestone-anxiety-rise-among-millennials-and-gen-z (accessed July 2024). This is a rise from 66 per cent of over 75s and 70 per cent of baby boomers who said that they felt this way when they were younger.

35 Faiza Mohammad, Nina Mill, and Kanak Ghosh, 'Marriages in England and Wales: 2019', ONS, 19 May 2022, available at: www.ons.gov.uk/peoplepopulationandcommunity/

birthsdeathsandmarriages/marriagecohabitationandcivil partnerships/bulletins/marriagesinenglandandwalesprovisional /2019 (accessed July 2024).

36 Ceri Roberts, 'The history of women and money', GoHenry, 7 March 2022, available at: www.gohenry.com/uk/blog/news/ the-history-of-women-and-money (accessed July 2024).

37 UK Parliament, 'Suffrage in wartime', UK Parliament, available at: www.parliament.uk/about/living-heritage/transformingsociety/ electionsvoting/womenvote/overview/suffragetteswartime (accessed July 2024).

38 Mildred A. Joiner and Clarence M. Weinger, 'Employment of women in war production', Bulletin, Reports and Analysis Division, Bureau of Employment Security, July 1942, available at: www.ssa. gov/policy/docs/ssb/v5n7/v5n7p4.pdf (accessed July 2024).

39 Women's Pioneer Housing (WPH), 'A history of WPH', WPH, n.d., available at: https://womenspioneer.co.uk/a-history-of-wph (accessed July 2024).

40 Dr Sundari Anitha and Professor Ruth Pearson, 'World War I: 1914–1918', Women and Work, Striking Women, available at: www.striking-women.org/module/women-and-work/world-war-i-1914-1918#:~:text=The%20women%20workers%20on%20 London,and%20ultimately%20won%20by%20women (accessed July 2024).

41 Hilary Spurling, 'The invisible women', *The Guardian,* 2 September 2007, available at: www.theguardian.com/ books/2007/sep/02/history.society (accessed July 2024).

42 Karen Harlow, '5 significant moments in the history of working women', CharityJob, 5 March 2024, available at: www.charityjob. co.uk/careeradvice/working-women/#:~:text=More%20 than%20a%20million%20women,and%20the%20work%20 was%20gruelling (accessed July 2024).

43 WPH, 'About us', WPH, n.d., available at: https://womenspioneer. co.uk/about-us (accessed July 2024).

44 WPH, 'A history of WPH', WPH, n.d.

45 Dr Sundari Anitha and Professor Ruth Pearson, 'World War II: 1939–1945', Women and Work, Striking Women, available at: www.striking-women.org/module/women-and-work/world-war-ii-1939-1945 (accessed July 2024).

46 Royal Institute of British Architects (RIBA), 'A dwelling of her own: Housing for single, working women in the 20th century', RIBA, n.d., available at: www.architecture.com/explore-architecture/inside-the-riba-collections/ a-dwelling-of-her-own-housing-for-working-women-in-the-20th-century (accessed July 2024).

47 Anitha and Pearson, 'World War II: 1939–1945'.

48 StudySmarter, 'Feminism in Britain (explanation)', StudySmarter app, n.d., available at: www.studysmarter.co.uk/explanations/history/modern-britain/feminism-in-britain (accessed July 2024).

49 Housing for Women, 'Our history', Housing for Women, n.d., available at: www.hfw.org.uk/about-us/who-we-are/our-history (accessed July 2024).

50 Paul Kerley, 'House-buyer time machine', BBC News, n.d., available at: www.bbc.co.uk/news/extra/pjfxZM72Gj/house-buyer-time-machine (accessed July 2024).

51 HM Land Registry, 'UK house price index', HM Land Registry, n.d., available at: https://landregistry.data.gov.uk/app/ukhpi/browse?from=1968-11-01&location=http%3A%2F%2Flandregistry.data.gov.uk%2Fid%2Fregion%2Flondon&to=2018-11-01&lang=en (accessed July 2024).

52 'Back when money was worth something', BBC News, 13 February 2001, available at: http://news.bbc.co.uk/1/hi/uk/1168149.stm (accessed July 2024).

53 Alice Duddy, 'International Women's Day: Women's rights to own property', HabitoHub, 1 June 2022, available at: www.habito.com/hub/article/international-womens-day-womens-rights-to-own-property#:~:text=But%20what%20about%20mortgages%3F,without%20facing%20discrimination%2C%20in%20theory (accessed July 2024).

54 Zach Wichter, 'The history of women and mortgages', Bankrate, 5 March 2024, available at: www.bankrate.com/mortgages/history-of-women-and-mortgages (accessed July 2024).

55 Mortgage Strategy, 'The female factor', Mortgage Strategy, 24 October 2005, available at: www.mortgagestrategy.co.uk/news/the-female-factor (accessed July 2024).

56 Craig Upright 'The converging gender wage gap 1980–2012', Contexts, Winter 2017, 16(1), pp. 72–4, available at: https://journals.sagepub.com   doifull/10.1177/1536504217696079#:~:text=As%20both%20the%20images%20and,for%20more%20than%20a%20decade (accessed July 2024).

57 Damian Grimshaw, Jill Robery, and Hugo Figueiredo, 'UK national report on the unadjusted and adjusted gender pay gap', European Commission's Expert Group on Gender and Employment, September 2002 available at: https://documents.manchester.ac.uk/display.aspx?DocID=50213#:~:text=From%20the%20early%201980s%20to,in%202001%20(Table%201.1) (accessed July 2024).

58 Kerley, 'House-buyer time machine'.

59 Woolf, *A Room of One's Own,* p. 22.

60 Duok, 'Pay gap, caring and confidence'.

61 Anna Boyles, 'Boston marriages and the queer history of women's suffrage', City of Boston,Mayor's Office, 15 November 2022, available at: www.boston.gov/news/boston-marriages-and-queer-history-womens-suffrage#:~:text=The%20term%20%E2%80%9CBoston%20Marriage%E2%80%9D%20refers,middle%20or%20upper%2Dclass%20women   (accessed July 2024).

2. Meeting point

1 Maya Angelou, 'One of Dr Maya Angelou's most important lessons', *The Oprah Winfrey Show,* 18 June 1997, available at: www.oprah.com/own-oprahshow/one-of-dr-maya-angelous-most-important-lessons_1 (accessed July 2024).

2 Kingfisher, 'How lockdown changed British attitudes towards

our home for good', Kingfisher, 9 September 2020, available at: www.kingfisher.com/en/media/news/kingfisher-news/2020/ how-lockdown-changed-british-attitudes-towards-our-homes- for-good.html (accessed July 2024).

3   R. I. M. Dunbar, 'Coevolution of neocortical size, group size and language in humans', *Behavoral and Brain Sciences,* December 1993, 16(4), pp. 681–94. For more on this see: www. bbc.com/future/article/20191001-dunbars-number-why-we- can-only-maintain-150-relationships (accessed July 2024).

4   Kelly Campbell, Nicole Holderness, and Matt Riggs, 'Friendship chemistry: An examination of underlying factors', *Social Science Journal,* June 2015, 52(2), pp. 239–47, available at: www.ncbi.nlm.nih.gov/pmc/articles/PMC4470381 (accessed July 2024).

5   K. H. Rogers and J. C. Biesanz, 'Knowing versus liking: Separating normative knowledge from social desirability in first impressions of personality, *Journal of Personality and Social Psychology,* 2015, 109(6), pp. 1105–16, available at: https:// psycnet.apa.org/doiLanding?doi=10.1037%2Fa0039587 (accessed July 2024).

6   Meg Jay, *The Defining Decade: Why your twenties matter and how to make the most of them now* (Edinburgh: Canongate Books, 2024).

3. Peas in a pod

1   Asia Lenae, 'Dolly Alderton on friendship as a more satisfying, everlasting form of love and how friendship metamorphoses', Asia Lenae's blog, available at: https://asialenae. com/2022/03/29/dolly-alderton-on-friendship-as-a-more- satisfying-everlasting-form-of-love-how-friendship- metamorphoses (accessed July 2024).

2   Renee Yaseen, 'Opinion: Why are Gen Zers valuing friendships over romance?', *Washington Post*, 21 September 2023, available at: www.washingtonpost.com/opinions/2023/09/21/postgrad-

relationship-hierarchy-friendships-romance (accessed July 2024).

3 R. I. M. Dunbar, 'Coevolution of neocortical size, group size and language in humans', *Behavoral and Brain Sciences,* December 1993, 16(4), pp. 681–94. For more on this see: www.bbc.com/future/article/20191001-dunbars-number-why-we-can-only-maintain-150-relationships (accessed July 2024).

4 Dr Ellyn Bader, 'A developmental model for healthy couples', Couples Institute, n.d., available at: www.couplesinstitute.com/a-developmental-model-for-healthy-couples (accessed July 2024).

5 Liz Steelman, '4 lessons to learn from people who moved in with their partners "way too early"', Apartment Therapy, available at: www.apartmenttherapy.com/cohabitating-early-expert-tips-36655763 (accessed July 2024).

6 Scott M. Stanley, Galena Kline Rhoades and Howard J. Markman, 'Sliding versus deciding: Inertia and premarital cohabitation effect', *Family Relations,* October 2006, 55(4), pp. 499–509, available at: https://onlinelibrary.wiley.com/doi/full/10.1111/j.1741-3729.2006.00418.x (accessed July 2024).

7 Julie Beck, 'How friendships change in adulthood: "We *need* to catch up soon!"', *The Atlantic,* 22 October 2015, available online at: www.theatlantic.com/health/archive/2015/10/how-friendships-change-over-time-in-adulthood/411466 (accessed July 2024).

8 Danielle Bayard Jackson, 'The rise of friendship therapy: A service for friends to navigate life changes and manage different communication styles', *Business Insider*, 19 August 2023, available at: www.businessinsider.com/friendship-therapy-why-it-works-repair-friendships-2023-8?r=US&IR=T#:~:text=Since%20the%20pandemic%2C%20the%20popularity,out%20this%20type%20of%20therapy (accessed July 2024).

9 Emily Langan, PhD, Faculty profiles, Wheaton College, see

under 'Research' at: www.wheaton.edu/academics/faculty/emily-langan (accessed July 2024).

4. Rupture and repair

1   Alain de Botton, 'On "rupture" and "repair", The School of Life, available at: www.theschooloflife.com/article/on-rupture-and-repair (accessed July 2024).

2   Andrew Grimmer, 'The cycle of rupture and repair in close relationships', Bristol CBT, 2019, available at: www.bristolcbt.co.uk/publications/the-cycle-of-rupture-and-repair-in-close-relationships (accessed July 2024).

3   Katie Shonk, '3 types of conflict and how to address them', Program on Negotiation, Harvard Law School blog, 23 April 2024, available at: www.pon.harvard.edu/daily/conflict-resolution/types-conflict (accessed July 2024).

4   Dr Ellyn Bader, 'A developmental model for healthy couples', Couples Institute, n.d., available at: www.couplesinstitute.com/a-developmental-model-for-healthy-couples (accessed July 2024).

5   Zoe Beaty, 'Generation rent: Stylist investigates the rising popularity of houseshares', Stylist, 2018, available at: www.stylist.co.uk/life/houseshares-pros-cons-having-flatmates-generation-rent/258346# (accessed July 2024).

6   Kuburic, S., *It's On Me: Accept hard truths, discover your self, and change your life* (New York: Dial Press, 2023), p. 156.

5. The pecking order

1   Gretchen Rubin, *Outer Order, Inner Calm: Declutter and organize to make more room for happiness* (London: Two Roads, 2020), p. xii.

2   'Role ambiguity' entry, ScienceDirect, available at: www.sciencedirect.com/topics/social-sciences/role-ambiguity (accessed July 2024).

3   Julia Samuel, *Every Family Has a Story: How to grow and move*

forward together (London: Penguin Life, 2022), p. 4.

4   Bernard A. Nijstad and Daan van Knippenberg, 'The psychology of groups: Basic principles, in Miles Hewston, Sofgan Strocbe and Klaus Jonas, *Introduction to Social Psychology: A European perspective,* 4th edn (Oxford: Blackwell, 2008), pp. 254–5, available at: www.blackwellpublishing.com/content/hewstonesocialpsychology/chapters/cpt12.pdf (accessed July 2024).

5   Vacuum cleaners.

6   Nijstad and van Knippenberg, 'The psychology of groups'.

7   Mike Robbins, *We're All in This Together: Creating a team culture of high performance, trust, and belonging* (London: Hay House, 2022).

8   Nijstad and van Knippenberg, 'The psychology of groups'.

9   Nijstad and van Knippenberg, 'The psychology of groups'.

10 Nijstad and van Knippenberg, 'The psychology of groups'.

11 Yi Han, Po Hao, Baiyin Yang and Wenxing Liu, 'How leaders' transparent behavior influences employee creativity: The mediating roles of psychological safety and ability to focus attention', *Journal of Leadership and Organizational Studies,* July 2017, 24(3), pp. 335–44, available at: www.researchgate.net/publication/319301490_How_Leaders'_Transparent_Behavior_Influences_Employee_Creativity (accessed July 2024).

6. Rental health

1   Matt Haig, *Reasons to Stay Alive* (Edinburgh: Canongate Books, 2015), p. 198.

2   Deloitte, 'Deloitte Gen Z and Millennial Survey: UK Gen Zs and Millennials reject employers who don't align with their values', Deloitte, 15 May 2024, available at: www.deloitte.com/uk/en/about/press-room/deloitte-genz-and-millennial-survey-uk-genzs-and-millennials-reject-employers-who-dont-align-with-their-values.html (accessed July 2024).

3   Thriving Center of Psychology, '2024 mental health outlook:

Growing demand for therapy among Gen Z and millennials', Thriving Center of Psychology blog, 19 December 2023, available at: https://thrivingcenterofpsych.com/blog/gen-z-millennial-therapy-statistics/#:~:text=2024%20Mental%20Health%20Plans,-Nearly%202%20in&text=Currently%2C%201%20in%205%20Gen,Depression (accessed July 2024).

4   Department for Levelling Up, Housing and Communities, 'Accredited official statistics: English Housing Survey 2021 to 2022: Private rented sector', Department for Levelling Up, Housing and Communities, 13 July 2023, available at: www.gov.uk/government/statistics/english-housing-survey-2021-to-2022-private-rented-sector/english-housing-survey-2021-to-2022-private-rented-sector#:~:text=23%25%20or%20990%2C000%20occupied%20private,%25%20or%202%20million%20dwellings (accessed July 2024).

5   Jihun Oh and Jeongseob Kim, 'Relationship between mental health and house sharing: Evidence from Seoul', *International Journal of Environmental Research and Public Health,* March 2021, 18(5), p. 2495, available at: www.ncbi.nlm.nih.gov/pmc/articles/PMC7967625/#B19-ijerph-18-02495 (accessed July 2024).

6   Tom Clark and Andrew Wenham, 'Anxiety nation?: Economic insecurity and mental distress in 2020s Britain', Joseph Rountree Foundation (JRF), November 2022, available at: www.jrf.org.uk/anxiety-nation-economic-insecurity-and-mental-distress-in-2020s-britain (accessed July 2024).

7   Oh and Kim, 'Relationship between mental health and house sharing'.

8   Dr Meg Arroll, *Tiny Traumas: When you don't know what's wrong, but nothing feels quite right* (London: Thorsons, 2023).

9   Pima Bakshi, 'Why are millennials and Gen Z the loneliest generations?', Refinery29, 12 October 2021, available at: www.refinery29.com/en-gb/millennial-gen-z-loneliness (accessed July 2024).

10   Jeffrey A. Hall and Andy J. Merolla, 'Connecting everyday talk

and time alone to global well-being', *Human Communication Research,* January 2020, 46(1), pp. 86–111, available at: https://academic.oup.com/hcr/article-abstract/46/1/86/5664814?redirectedFrom=fulltext (accessed July 2024).

7. Precious things

1 William Morris, 'The beauty of life', talk delivered at the Birmingham Society of Arts and School of Design, 19 February 1810, *Hopes and Fears for Art* (London: Ellis & White, 1882), Chapter 3.

2 Christian Jarrett, 'The psychology of stuff and things', *The Psychologist,* 13 August 2013, available at: www.bps.org.uk/psychologist/psychology-stuff-and-things (accessed July 2024).

3 Jarrett, 'The psychology of stuff and things'.

4 Jarrett, 'The psychology of stuff and things'.

5 Jane Kroger and Vivienne Adair, 'Symbolic meaning of valued personal objects in identity transitions of late adulthood', *Identity,* January 2008, 8(1), pp. 5–24, available at: www.researchgate.net/publication/233286580_Symbolic_Meanings_of_Valued_Personal_Objects_in_Identity_Transitions_of_Late_Adulthood (accessed July 2024).

6 University of Chicago Press Journals, 'In children and adolescents, low self-esteem increases materialism', ScienceDaily, 16 November 2007, available at: www.sciencedaily.com/releases/2007/11/071112133809.htm (accessed July 2024).

7 Jarrett, 'The psychology of stuff and things'.

8 Eugene Halton, *The Great Brain Suck: And other American epiphanies* (Chicago, IL: University of Chicago Press, 2008), p. 206.

8. Dating by committee

1 Gerald Martin, *Gabriel García Márquez: A life* (London: Bloomsbury, 2008), p. 229.

2 Dr Ellyn Bader, 'Stepping stones to intimacy: A positive

outlook on problems', Couples Institute, n.d., available at: www.couplesinstitute.com/stepping-stones-to-intimacy-a-positive-outlook-on-problems-in-couples-relationships (accessed July 2024).

It's time

1   Brené Brown, 'Manifesto of the brave and brokenhearted', *Rising Strong* (London: Vermilion, 2015), pp. 267–8.

2   Index Digital Team, 'Moving house ranked "most stressful life event" by 57% of Brits', Index Digital, 14 February 2023, available at: www.indexdigital.co.uk/home-gardens/moving-house-ranked-most-stressful-life-event-by-57-of-brits (accessed July 2024).

3   Patrick Collinson, 'The other generation rent: Meet the people flatsharing in their 40s', *The Guardian,* 25 September 2015, available at: www.theguardian.com/money/2015/sep/25/flatsharing-40s-housing-crisis-lack-homes-renting-london (accessed July 2024).

4   Dinsa Sachan, 'The broken hearts club', *The Psychologist,* 7 August 2018, available at: www.bps.org.uk/psychologist/broken-hearts-club (accessed July 2024).

5   Dr Henry Cloud, *Necessary Endings: The employees, businesses, and relationships that all of us have to give up in order to move forward* (New York: HarperBusiness, 2011), p. 227.

6   Leonie Koban, Ethan Kross, Choong-Wan Woo, Luka Ruzic, and Tor D. Wagner, 'Frontal-brainstem pathways mediating placebo effects on social rejection', *Journal of Neuroscience,* 29 March 2017, 37(13), pp. 3621–31, available at: www.jneurosci.org/content/37/13/3621 (accessed July 2024).

7   Dr Becca Bland, 'The living loss: Family estrangement and stages of grief', Dr Becca Bland, 25 July 2023, available at: www.beccabland.com/post/the-living-loss-family-estrangement-stages-of-grief (accessed July 2024).

Select bibliography

Arroll, Dr M., *Tiny Traumas: When you don't know what's wrong, but nothing feels quite right* (London: Thorsons, 2023).

Cloud, Dr H., *Necessary Endings: The employees, businesses, and relationships that all of us have to give up in order to move forward* (New York: HarperBusiness, 2011).

Cohen, C., *BFF?: The truth about female friendship* (London: Penguin, 2023).

Csikszentmihalyi, M., and Rochberg-Halton, E., *The Meaning of Things: Domestic symbols and the self* (Cambridge University Press, 1981).

Day, E., *Friendaholic: Confessions of a friendship addict* (London: 4th Estate, 2024).

Friedman, A., and Sow, A., *Big Friendship: How we keep each other close* (New York: Simon & Schuster, 2021).

Jay, Dr M., *The Defining Decade: Why your twenties matter and how to make the most of them now* (Edinburgh: Canongate Books, 2024).

Kuburic, S., *It's On Me: Accept hard truths, discover your self, and change your life* (New York: Dial Press, 2023).

Reed Turrell, E., *Please Yourself: How to stop people-pleasing and transform the way you live* (London: 4th Estate, 2021).

Samuel, J., *Every Family Has a Story: How to grow and move forward together* (London: Penguin Life, 2022).

About the author

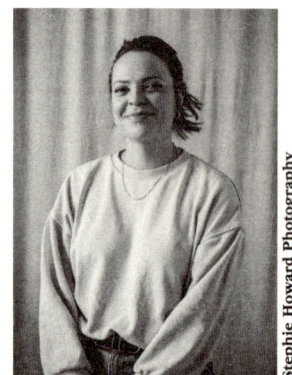

Stephie Howard Photography

Alice Wilkinson is a writer, editor and journalist at *The Telegraph*. A previous editor of Waitrose Health, her writing has been featured in many national newspapers and magazines. In 2019 Alice was shortlisted for the Professional Publishers Award (PPA) for Writer of the Year. The following year, she was selected as one of the PPA's 30 Under 30. In 2022, she was shortlisted for the British Society of Magazine Editor's New Editor of The Year. Today, Alice writes a Substack newsletter titled 'Addressing' where she explores house sharing, home and belonging.